T0248205

NO ONE GETS TO FALL APART

NO ONE GETS

TO FALL APART

A Memoir

Sarah LaBrie

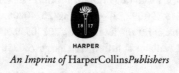

HARPER

An Imprint of HarperCollins*Publishers*

This is a work of nonfiction. The events and experiences detailed
herein are all true and have been faithfully rendered as I have
remembered them, to the best of my ability. Some names, identities, and
circumstances have been changed in order to protect the integrity and/or
privacy of the various individuals involved.

Though conversations come from my keen recollection of them, they are
not written to represent word-for-word documentation; rather, I've retold
them in a way that evokes the real feeling and meaning of what was said in
keeping with the true essence of the mood and spirit of the event.

HarperCollins books may be purchased for educational, business, or
sales promotional use. For information, please email the Special Markets
Department at SPsales@harpercollins.com.

FIRST EDITION

Designed by Bonni Leon-Berman

Library of Congress Cataloging-in-Publication Data

Names: LaBrie, Sarah, author.
Title: No one gets to fall apart / Sarah LaBrie.
Description: First edition. | New York, NY: Harper, 2024.
Identifiers: LCCN 2023053924 (print) | LCCN 2023053925 (ebook) |
ISBN 9780063280724 (hardcover) | ISBN 9780063280748 (ebook)
Subjects: LCSH: LaBrie, Sarah. | Children of the mentally ill—United States—
Biography. | Mentally ill—United States—Biography. | Mentally ill—Family
relationships—United States. | Mothers and daughters—United States.
Classification: LCC RC464.L33 A3 2024 (print) | LCC RC464.L33
(ebook) | DDC 616.890092 [B]—dc23/eng/20240708
LC record available at https://lccn.loc.gov/2023053924
LC ebook record available at https://lccn.loc.gov/2023053925

24 25 26 27 28 LBC 5 4 3 2 1

For Justin, Kim, Monica, and Joan

It dawned on me that all these assertive, grown-up people who had just been talking and laughing were going about bent over, occupied with something invisible; that they conceded something was there that they could not see.

—*Rainer Maria Rilke,* The Notebooks of Malte Laurids Brigge

NO ONE GETS TO FALL APART

ONE

IN MARCH 2017, MY GRANDMOTHER in Houston calls me in Los Angeles to tell me my mother was recently found on the side of the freeway, parked, honking her horn, her car filled with notes in which she outlined federal agents' plans to kill her. In the car was a receipt for bottled water from George Bush Intercontinental Airport, over an hour away. Later we learned she spent the day there terrified she was going to be murdered, hoping if something happened it would be caught on a security camera.

Actually, my grandmother informs me, my mother has been saying cars driven by sunglasses-wearing white men have been chasing her down the highway since February. The number started at ten, then rose to dozens and then to hundreds. She called and wrote notes to my grandmother's friends and colleagues, to neighbors, to strangers, detailing her persecution, leading the police to appear more than once at her home.

At times my mother was so afraid she slept in her car, not going inside to shower or change. She was fired from her nursing job after she drowned her work laptop in the bathtub. She purchased cameras to take pictures of the people following her then threw the cameras away. She took my aunt Tina on walks through the neighborhood and pointed out all the white cars. "See?" she said. "How they all have their lights on in the daytime?" My aunt tried to tell her the lights were a feature of the cars and not an element of some conspiracy, but my mother did not believe her.

She was committed to the psychiatric ward at Bayshore Medical Center, a hospital outside the city. The hospital called Aunt Tina, who called my grandmother, who tried to get her released the following morning but was not allowed to see or speak to her. Nurses injected her with medication that put her to sleep for forty-eight hours. When she woke up, she called my grandmother and asked, "What happened? Who said someone wanted to kill me?" My grandmother and Aunt Tina told her the truth, which was that nobody aside from my mother herself believed anyone wanted to kill her.

Since coming home from the hospital, my grandmother tells me, my mother is back to normal, looking for a new nursing job. She blames the Houston traffic and the onset of menopause. She says the psychiatrist who released her diagnosed her as severely depressed.

I hang up awash in guilt, open the calendar on my phone, and try to remember what I was doing for the nights she was in the hospital and I didn't know. A friend directed a Schubert performance by the Los Angeles Philharmonic that I wanted to go to but ultimately skipped in favor of working on the novel I'd been trying to finish for years. I was home writing and feeling bad about not going to the symphony while my mother was in a car on the side of the highway begging someone to save her life. I remember an odd phone conversation with her the week before last; she called to apologize for something she once said that hurt me. It was the first time we'd spoken in a while, and that phone call combined with this new information suggests conclusions I don't feel quite ready to accept.

"WHY ARE YOU ON THE floor?" Ethan, my boyfriend, asks that night when he comes home. He has a mild form of obsessive-compulsive personality disorder, and my sitting on the ground with my phone in my hand appears to offend him. I can't answer. What my grandmother said about the cars and the notes and the police appears so absurd, I feel certain he'll laugh or he won't understand or I won't be able to find the words to describe what happened at all.

"My mother's acting weird," I say. I repeat my grandmother's story.

"You know, paranoia is also a form of narcissism," he says. He turns on the TV and the living room fills with the sounds of the L.A. Clippers blowing another fourth-quarter lead. "You know how your mom is," he adds. "Sometimes she acts out."

"I don't think she was acting out." I slide up the wall. "The police found her. She didn't go to them."

"All I'm saying is, she hasn't always been a very good mother to you," Ethan replies, and even though this is true, I'm not sure how it makes a difference. In the kitchen, I pour myself a glass of honey-colored wine and as I do, I feel the left side of my face go numb. The numbness travels down my left arm and into my hand. I wonder if the fact that my mother has succumbed to psychosis is making my body believe it can, too. If my mind believes it is free to do whatever it wants without me, then who am I to stop it? What do I stop it with?

THE MORNING AFTER MY GRANDMOTHER calls, I open my novel manuscript and stare at it. The situation seems hopeless. Some of it is good and some of it is bad and nothing I do, short of starting from scratch, will make the bad parts better. I open a new version and try editing out the bad parts and am left with nothing but fragments. I close the document, open a browser, and spend the next twenty minutes combing through lists of productivity hacks on Reddit.

My mother calls. I pick up and she starts talking before I can say hello. She says, "I heard your voice. It seemed like you said, 'Mom, you have to get up, you have to go listen to the radio.' And then I got up and listened to the radio. The people on the radio said your name. Everywhere I go, the names are so familiar."

She tells me she's stuck on a game show and being surveilled from an airplane in the sky. She thinks the surveillance might have something to do with Facebook, because people are always using their phones. "Facebook or one of those TV shows like *The Bachelorette*," she says. She saw on a magazine cover when she was at the grocery store a story about a millionaire who was looking to marry someone. An actor. He used to be married to this really pretty Australian lady? They're not married anymore.

"Tom Cruise?" I ask. Yes, she says. Tom Cruise.

She saw Tom Cruise on a magazine cover and he was looking for someone to marry and she thinks the game show she is trapped in has to do with marriage, relationships, and money. She's being held hostage and whenever she goes out, she feels like people are looking at her. Like, they look at her, then look down at their phones? She knows it sounds crazy, but every time she tries to do something—

"Let me put it this way," my mother says. "My car is totaled. I try to take the bus, but I get lost. I ask someone for directions, and they send me the opposite way and I have to ask someone else. I don't know what's happening because I'm not on the internet. Even when I had a laptop, I couldn't look directions up because my laptop was being held hostage."

Then she finishes all in a rush: A man named Lance Blanks is holding her hostage. He is the only person she's ever known in her life who has money, who could get in an airplane and hang out in the sky and watch her. She thinks Lance Blanks is the reason she feels a pinprick in her foot when she says certain names. "Like now," she says. "Something's pricking my foot. And look, I'm getting pricked again!"

Lance Blanks is a former professional basketball player. He played for the Detroit Pistons and retired in 1999. He and my mother went to the same high school in Houston for a while and were once friends. They'd fallen out of touch. But I can remember a night they had dinner when he was passing through town. She sounded tremendously happy to have seen him.

Now she wants me to listen out for Lance's name. She wants to know if that same sensation of being pricked happens to me. She wants to tell me she has these strange jolts in her fingers. "Why is this happening?" she keeps asking. "Why is this happening to me?" At any point, I think, she's going to reveal she's only joking. I wait. She doesn't. After making me promise not to tell my grandmother what she's told me, she hangs up.

I go outside and walk up and down the narrow sidewalk between my building and the one next door, searching the sky for planes. My friend Melissa, an architect who lives one apartment over with her boyfriend, tends the vegetable garden she's cultivating in our tiny parking lot. She wiggles her hand in front of my nose, showing me her new engagement ring. "When do you think Ethan's going to propose?" she asks. "How long have you guys been together? Six years?" My phone vibrates. My grandmother calling. I wave at Melissa without answering her question and walk away.

"She totaled her car?" I say into the phone. My grandmother confirms this is correct and the world swings around me in a loop, my heart beating so hard I have to double over to get it to stop. It feels like a screw got caught in my chest and is winding its way deeper in. I reach and reach for a revelation, an epiphany, a way out of this story, but no revelation appears.

"You look at the car and wonder how a person survived that," my grandmother says, her voice tight. "She went through an intersection at a yellow light. She said the other car came out of nowhere. She asked the other driver repeatedly if they were hurt, and the person said no."

I ask my grandmother what my mother is doing right now.

"Looking at a piece of art, a painting she keeps in her room," she says. "There's a stroke on that painting she doesn't understand. She thinks somebody came in and put it there."

Ethan comes up the sidewalk weighed down with farmers' market produce. Our dog, Larry Bird, trails behind him. I hurry off the phone to help.

"Stop looking like that," he says as he unloads bags into my arms.

"Like what?"

"You look so scared."

I'm thinking about a story my mother told me once about the son of one of her patients, who had a psychotic break. He shot a crow off the power line outside his house with a BB gun, brought it inside, dipped it in flour, and tried to fry it. He said he was making his sister lunch. I'm imagining an illness that could do something like that spreading its way through my mother and turning her into someone I don't recognize, and then I'm imagining it making its way through her into me.

...

I NEVER FEEL more like my mother than when Ethan is driving and I'm in the passenger seat. That weekend, we're on the way to a wedding in wine country with the dog. Ethan keeps taking his eyes off the road to look at the map on his phone, and I'm certain he is going to swerve into traffic. "I swear to God, you're getting on my last goddamn nerve!" I shout and hear her voice in my mouth.

"Jesus Christ. I'm sorry," Ethan says, turning to look at me as he apologizes. "Could you stop yelling?"

"Look at the road!" I yell. A boy on a bicycle speeds past us, narrowly missing our bumper.

I get a text from my grandmother saying my mother seemed agitated at lunch, that she kept the receipt from their meal as evidence in case strangers were trying to poison her. Then, Aunt Tina texts to say she took my mother to buy a new camera to photograph the white men in sunglasses she believes follow her everywhere. Now, they both say, she listens to Christian music on the radio all day long. Babbie Mason. Shannon Wexelberg. Larnelle Harris. Religious singers whose names I have to look up. A friend of my grandmother who stops by often to visit has taken to calling her "The Holy One."

Ethan and I pull off in a town called Lost Hills ("Pop. 1938," reads the sign that leads us off the highway) so the dog can pee, and I have an idea for a short story. The story is about a couple like Ethan and me. The girlfriend discovers her mother is losing her mind. The following weekend, the girlfriend and the boyfriend go on a road trip to a wedding. On the drive up, the girlfriend starts to believe her boyfriend is plotting against her. Their car breaks down in a town called Lost Hills, and creepy things start to happen: an airplane appears to be following them, a man holding a camera takes a picture of them as they pass, and a boy on a bike drives directly into the car so it looks as though they've hit him. The town police come and question the boyfriend and girlfriend separately. She thinks the boyfriend was betraying her, telling lies about her to the police, and it turns out he was.

The girl gets tied up, jailed, tortured. At the end of the story, we learn none of what the girl believes is real. She's been institutionalized the entire time, and her mother is coming to visit her. In the final scenes, the mother has the same conversation with the daughter they had on the phone at the beginning, only now we see they are in a hospital, the mother apologizing to her daughter, the girl, locked in her own head, unable to understand.

I write the idea down in my phone before it can disintegrate. I study the words on my screen. I wonder if what they mean is I want to trade places with my mother. To stop whatever is happening to her by changing things around so it is happening to me. Or if what they mean is what comes for her will inevitably come for us both.

The dog pees by the road. We get back in the car. We leave Lost Hills and drive to Paso Robles. All the way there and then in the bedroom at our Airbnb, I refresh the news on my phone. Donald Trump bombed Syria. North Korea has functional nuclear weapons. Starbucks is making a unicorn-flavored drink. Bill O'Reilly is losing his TV show due to sexual harassment allegations but is already planning a comeback in the form of a podcast. I check *New York* magazine and the *Washington Post*. Every time I come up for air and remember what is happening to her, it's like finding out for the first time all over again. I refresh and refresh. I scroll and scroll. If I had been in regular contact with her. If I had been nicer. If I called her when she wanted me to, no matter how mean she was or how busy I got. I reread the text message she sent me last Mother's Day, left unanswered because we weren't speaking: Happy Mother's Day to me!! Maybe if I'd written back, none of this would be happening now.

...

THE UBER DRIVER WHO PICKS us up from our Airbnb to take us to the rehearsal dinner has strobe lights in his car. He offers us candy for answering trivia questions. Where is the sea of tranquility? The moon. What are the names of Michael Jackson's three children? Paris, Blanket, and Prince. What is the best-selling album of all time? *Thriller*. What was the first video MTV ever played? "Video Killed the Radio Star." I get a Blow Pop for knowing the answers. The driver coasts along the side of a mountain, and I feel sure we are going to fall. "If we die, who will take care of the dog?" I whisper to Ethan. We've left her behind at the rental.

"The dog will be fine," he says and squeezes my hand.

Our Uber driver tells us his own dogs' names are Janis and Turner, after Janis Joplin and Tina Turner, and he loves them more than his kids. He tells us he's been married to his wife for twenty-two years and he doesn't know what she does for a living but she looks damn good going to work. He talks about the snowpack and how Mammoth will have skiing through July because of all the recent rain after years and years of drought. My mother's sickness could be like the droughts that plague California. It could come and go and come and go and come back worse every time.

At the rehearsal dinner, I sit next to Ethan's friend from film school whose father is about to die of cancer. The father is bedridden, his mind addled. Ethan's friend lists his symptoms casually, and I feel put off by his nonchalance before I understand. This is what Ethan was trying to tell me: no one is allowed to fall apart.

Under a tent, various meats lie spread out on wood blocks surrounded by fruit and seeds and nuts. The tent is filled with trees and flowers strung with lights. I take a glass of champagne from a passing tray. I want my mother to have the life I have. To drink champagne at a wedding on a farm. Her own wedding to my dad took place shortly after they met as students at San Francisco State University in a park in East Oakland. She was nineteen and pregnant with me. Afterward they went to my dad's parents' little house in Las Palmas to eat.

Ethan and I spot a hedge funder we know, one of the groom's best friends. We cross the floor to say hello. "Do you two ever want to get married?" he asks us. His tall, blond date stares at us, blue eyes wide. We take sips from our glasses and nod and smile and pretend we can't hear him over the music, then dance away. *My mom is broken*, my mind sings. *My mom is broken. My mom is fucking broken.*

The next day after the ceremony, the bride and groom do the hora, and Ethan asks me if I've ever seen anything like it before. People are always asking me this question at Jewish weddings because I am Black, but I never expected one of these people to be my boyfriend. But then the bride's dad gives a speech about how much the bride and groom belong together predicated on their shared love of triathlons and hang gliding and Ethan and I laugh inappropriately at the exact same time and I remember why we chose each other.

"So, when are you planning to pop the question?" the groom's father asks Ethan. Next to him, the groom's mother beams. Ethan looks at me, then looks away. I look down at my hands. Neither one of us responds. I'm thinking about the only other delusional person I've met, a racist cab driver who drove me haphazardly from Park Slope to Penn Station and told me he owned all the skyscrapers we passed.

On stage, our drunk friend slurs the words to "Satisfaction" while the band plays along. If I were a different person, I think, dancing, maybe my mother would still be sane. The groom leads a parade up to the main house, then goes inside with his new wife, leaving us to return, alone, to the party. It occurs to me that my mother is almost certainly going to kill herself out of fear. The thought makes me feel heavy and tired.

Back at the Airbnb that night, a storm passes over the city. Gusts of wind push up against the windows. Ethan stretches out on the bed, closes his eyes, and rolls onto his side. I press my body into his and the way it feels reminds me that I am an animal who once lived in a pack, surrounded by fur and heat.

...

MY GRANDMOTHER CALLS to tell me the state Board of Nursing is requiring my mother to undergo psychological testing to determine whether she is still capable of doing her job. If she doesn't pass the psychiatric evaluation, she may have her nursing license taken away.

"Whatever they gave her at the hospital seems to be working. I think she can at least get herself food to eat and change the oil in her car and pay her bills. Whereas before, she was so paranoid . . ."

I'm thinking about the last conversation I had with her. About her terror of Lance Blanks. Of his plane in the sky watching her. Of Tom Cruise.

"It didn't sound like things were better. It sounds like she needs help—"

"No. No," my grandmother says. "If she can get herself through this nursing board inquiry, she'll be okay. She can start work again. All she needs is some stability. And for that, she has to have money."

I try to keep frustration from creeping into my voice without success. "But that's what I'm saying. She doesn't have money because she quit her job because she's sick. She needs help from a professional."

In 2014, I went home to attend my cousin's high school graduation and found the family dog, Chacha, covered in fleas. That year, my cousin was dating a mean girl, a habitual liar who had briefly convinced my cousin to run away to Florida, sparking a weekend of crisis. After graduation, my cousin was also planning to attend a mediocre college in New Orleans, even though they'd been offered a full ride to a more selective school in Atlanta. My grandmother and Aunt Tina were afraid of the choices my cousin was making, but seemed to not want to talk about it with me or them or with each other, and the stress of not talking about it was leading to the neglect of the dog. When I raised a commotion, my grandmother shushed me, as if the problem was that I might be overheard by a neighbor rather than that the dog's fur was infested so badly she could barely move.

"Your mother can manage on her own," my grandmother insists now. "It would be nice if she could join some kind of support group, I guess, but she has to have a job first. She has to be able to eat and pay her car insurance. Practical concerns."

...

THE FOLLOWING WEEK, MY MOTHER drives herself to her psychiatric evaluation and does not come back. The hospital calls my grandmother to tell her the police found her parked in the middle of a busy street. She heard a voice on her way to the appointment that told her she didn't have to go. Now she's in the hospital again.

"So it's exactly like the other time," says my weary grandmother. "But this time it's even harder to understand because, before, she was under severe stress. Now, I could see if something was really wrong with her. Really serious, schizophrenia or something—"

"You don't think it sounds a little bit like schizophrenia?"

"There's so much mental illness around, it's unbelievable," my grandmother acquiesces vaguely. "But your mother is sane. She's perfectly sane. She's able to work. She's able to drive."

I hear myself say, "Should I come home?"

"No, no, no, no," my grandmother says. A descending scale. "We're taking it step-by-step. She's going to be fine."

BACK IN 2014, I REMEMBER leaving my cousin's high school graduation ceremony in my mother's white Toyota Corolla. In the back seat was a pile of garbage: a table leg, a dented filing cabinet, and a stack of Xerox paper loose in a plastic bag, blinding in the sunlight.

"What's all this?" I asked.

"I'm moving into the spare rooms in Granny's office," she said. "I'm leaving Jerome." She made a frustrated noise. "That reminds me. I have to go downtown. To the courthouse. He made me change my last name and now I want to change it back."

All I knew about Jerome, her soon to be ex-husband, was that he worked at the port of Houston unloading shipping containers. I didn't even know where in the city they lived together. Soon, it will become clear that her marriage to this stranger—a con-man who gets two other women pregnant in the time they are together and who ultimately disappears from her life as abruptly as he enters it—was an early sign of her decompensation. But at the time, I only wondered if my grandmother and Aunt Tina knew she'd changed her last name, and if it would have made a difference if they had. Back then, we took her sudden marriage the way we took all the strange things she did, in stride. Now I think that our reactions to her behavior were not entirely unlike the reactions of my grandmother and Aunt Tina to my cousin and to the flea-bitten dog. In our family, though we loved and wanted the best for each other, it was policy to let fate take each person where it would, even if doing so meant failing to avert disaster.

TWO

WILLIAM JAMES BELIEVED IT WAS impossible to study human consciousness without studying the connections between people. Franz Kafka writes that every person, even the emptiest, is, if one will only look carefully, the center of a tight circle that forms about him here and there.[1] Neuropsychiatrist Dan Siegel suggests we build ourselves out of our understanding of our childhoods as we're convinced they happened and not as they took place. Stories, Siegel writes, determine the course of our lives, especially when it comes to our relationships with our own children.[2] So far as the self exists, it is recursive, constantly forming and reforming according to what we tell ourselves about the past.

German philosopher and critic Walter Benjamin wrote, "Origin, although a thoroughly historical category, nonetheless has nothing to do with beginnings. . . . The term origin does not mean the process of becoming of that which has emerged, but much more, that which emerges out of the process of becoming and disappearing."[3]

My senior year of college, I took a course on Benjamin taught by a professor who had published a co-translation of his epic, collagic history of modern Paris, *The Arcades Project*. Benjamin wrote *The Arcades Project* in part by drawing together excerpts from primary sources so that sense emerged from their arrangement rather than directly from the texts themselves. His method felt revolutionary when I first encountered it, at once both entirely new and intensely familiar.

The novel I'm trying to write, *The Anatomy Book*, is about a fictional philosopher named Nicholas Canton, who is based on Walter Benjamin, attempting to find the key to time travel. I'm writing it in part due to my infatuation with Benjamin and in part because I'm still haunted by my inability to pass that professor's course. I'd thought of myself, up until 2007, as a smart, ambitious person blessed with the ability to finish what I started. But now, that version of me was gone. Every page of the final paper I couldn't complete exposed the chasm between what I believed about myself and reality. Finally, that spring, having descended into this divide, I dropped first the Benjamin class then all my classes, one by one.

A core tenet of schizophrenia—the disorder with which my mother will eventually be officially diagnosed—is the difficulty patients have when it comes to resolving threads of incoming sensory perception. Sufferers believe listening devices have been inserted into their teeth or surveillance cameras placed throughout their homes. My mother, in the midst of these delusions, persists in asking: *Why me? Why now? Why this?* That final year of college, skipping the classes I needed to pass to graduate but, at the same time, unable to bring myself to get out of bed and go, my questions were the same. *Why me? Why now? Why this?*

For several months in 1935 and again in 1936, Benjamin conducted research for the Arcades Project in the Cabinet des Estampes at the Bibliothèque Nationale. There he collected and categorized images he thought epitomized Paris at the start of the modern era. A faded poster. A gas lamp. An exhibition catalog for the 1939 World's Fair. He believed it was only in these "concrete, 'small, particular moments'" that "the origins of the present could be found,"[4] and in these origins the answer to the questions: *Why us, why now, why this*?

In the story of my mother and me, a first image would be the Toyota Celica she drove when I was small pulling into our driveway, her finger pointing at the immense flocks of blackbirds perched on the power lines above us. I am five. She is twenty-five, unassumingly small, often harried. She smiles rarely, but when she does, she is extremely pretty.

"If you're bad," she tells me, "the birds will know. They'll give you a paintbrush, and you'll have to paint the sky black at night. You'll paint and paint. You'll never get the chance to sleep."

"Why won't I sleep?" I ask her, delighted, knowing the answer.

"Because as soon as you're done, they'll make you wash the paint off so it's day again. You'll have to start over!"

"And what if I won't?" I ask. "What if I say no?"

"Then they'll come in through the window at night and smother you." I imagine feathers against my skin, the sound of rustling black wings.

We live in a fourplex in Third Ward owned by my grandmother, who runs her small natural health care business out of the largest unit and rents the others out. I have my own bunk bed in our apartment's one bedroom, but my mother and I sleep next to each other in the living room on the foldout couch. Sometimes as my mother falls asleep, she rolls away, and I grow desperate for her voice.

"Don't go to bed yet," I say. "Tell me about the shipwreck."

My favorite bedtime story is a story she saw on the news about a man and a woman whose boat capsized in shark-infested waters. The man died, and the woman had to drink her own pee to survive. Because pee, she explains to me—she's still in nursing school and likes to share with me everything she learns—is sterile. "Now close your eyes. Even if you can't sleep, close your eyes and lie there with your eyes closed, okay?"

I do as she says then open them to find she's turned away again. I shake her awake in abject despair.

"What?"

"If you sleep like that, I won't have a beautiful face to look at."

And though she shushes me again, she will repeat the compliment for years.

My mother works hospital shifts at night, but even when we are both home during the day, the apartment sometimes fills with a silence like a fog that won't lift. I find her sitting on the edge of her bed, staring into space. She appears extremely lonely, and her loneliness makes me feel lonely too. I try to force her gaze into mine. "Say something," I say.

"Something."

"No, say *something*."

"Something."

I'm scream-laughing, but she is not. And on and on like this, the silence not broken by the noise I make but growing thicker because of it.

HOUSTON WEATHER IS HURRICANE WEATHER. Thunder bellows like an enormous heartbeat. Lightning flashes so bright it makes nighttime look like day. My mother sits on a stool above me and combs out my hair while rain hammers the windows. I lean back into her knees. We're watching the sitcom *Martin* on her little TV on the floor. Pam, Martin's nemesis, calls him an idiot. My mother laughs.

"What's an idiot?" I ask.

"A stupid person," my mother says.

"Mama, you're an idiot," I say. I laugh. Her attacks, like Houston storms, emerge fully formed out of what moments before appeared to be a cloudless sky. It's hard to know how mad she is going to be until it's much too late. After she hits me, she puts me in the closet and shuts the door. On a shelf, I keep two turquoise marbles with chimes inside that Aunt Tina brought me home from a trip to Las Vegas. She's taught me to roll their cool surfaces over each other, and I do this in the dark for half an hour until my mother lets me out.

A SECOND IMAGE: A PHOTOGRAPH in the *Marshall News Messenger* from 1966 of my grandmother in a shiny beehive hairdo looking like a homecoming queen.[5] Beneath the photograph, an article lauding her for graduating with highest honors from Pemberton High School in the East Texas town of Marshall.

A different photograph, published twelve years later in *Ebony* magazine, shows my grandmother at thirty-three. She's seated behind a desk in gold hoops, a collared silk shirt, and a scarf tied beneath her tidy Afro. The caption describes her as an attorney and the director of Houston's Fair Housing Division. The headline reads "Houston: Golden City of Opportunity." "For young Blacks with skills," a local official is quoted as saying about my grandmother's generation, "this is the city of the 21st Century."[6]

After her own mother, Alma, died of breast cancer, my grandmother, then forty-two, underwent a spiritual awakening. She took courses on Buddhism and spent weekends at ashrams and read all of Carlos Castaneda and Krishnamurti. She stopped eating meat, started doing yoga, and studied holistic healing. She left her job as an attorney and opened her natural health care office along with a bookstore dedicated to African history. She called the bookstore Sankofa, after a Ghanaian letterform from the Twi language that takes the shape of a bird with its head curved backward and translates to "go back and get it."

In this way, she became the perpetually composed naturopath I remember working out of the many-roomed office space downstairs from our apartment. In these rooms are shelves of medical textbooks, a full-sized replica skeleton, heating pads, and sensors covered in menthol gel. Books from the bookstore, which closed a few years after it opened, line the hallways: first editions of *Just Above My Head* by James Baldwin, *And the Walls Came Tumbling Down* by Ralph David Abernathy, *Going to the Territory* by Ralph Ellison. A different room holds a glass cabinet full of Africana: porcelain saltshakers in the shape of old mammies wearing painted red-and-white smiles, little Black boys eating watermelon and grinning, Aunt Jemima corn meal boxes, a terrifying rag doll with a white girl's face on one side and a Black enslaved girl's face on the other. She says they recall a history that needs to be remembered. My grandmother is fixated on history, on inheritance, on what we do and don't recall. On summer breaks, she brings my mother, Aunt Tina, and me with her on trips to Ghana, to Mali, to South Africa. We visit the Elmina Castle slave depot in Cape Coast. On a different trip, I befriend a boy my age who lives in a Dogon village in Timbuktu.

I turn fourteen on vacation in Accra and, over dinner at the hotel, everyone in our travel group sings me "Happy Birthday." Someone takes a picture. When we get home, I show it to my mother. "You're so hateful," she says to me matter-of-factly, examining the photograph, then looking up at me to see how I'll react. She's right that my smile in the photo is fake. I didn't want anyone to sing to me. I dislike being the center of attention. I'm scared of her, not only because she is angry all the time now but because she knows me well enough to see everything I'm trying to hide and will not hesitate to deploy this knowledge to hurt me. I take the picture back and walk away.

My grandmother suspects my mother inherited her now almost constant state of rage from my grandfather Vernon, a violent man whom she divorced when my mother was five, and who was either murdered or committed suicide by the time my mother was fourteen, dead from asphyxiation under a Lincoln Continental in the garage of the gas station he owned. She also says her own mother, Alma, who spent most of her time in bed and was likely depressed before anyone used the word, may have passed down difficult genes. If only my mother would choose to be aware of her inheritance, my grandmother says, if only she chose to look inward, she might figure out how to feel better.

But when I ask my grandmother to elaborate on her own past—to tell me what happened to her when she was a student in the 1960s living in the still de facto segregated dorms at University of Texas, for example—she only wants to talk about her best friend at the time, Maudie, who taught her how to take care of my mother when she was an infant, and Maudie's husband, who, after college, partnered with my grandfather to open a nightclub, which, in turn, was how my grandmother learned to operate a business. It is important to my grandmother that I understand life is not shaped in any way that is important by forces outside our control. That, armed with a healthy dose of self-awareness, every person gets to decide, in one way or another, who they will be and what kind of life they will lead.

The idea that I might inherit what my mother inherited from her father scares me, but I'm comforted by the idea that my grandmother has been able to overcome what her own mother, who she says hardly ever got out of bed except to beat her, handed down to her through sheer force of will. Of course, I know now there is a difference between having a temper and having mental illness, but back then I still thought it was all a matter of control.

But then, on a trip to Milan with my grandmother, I wander off in a train station, distracted by the ornate ceiling. When she finds me after a frantic search, she lunges at me. I shout in surprise and fall backward, trying to explain. She shoves me down a second time, insisting I listen to her and stop talking back. I run into a bathroom to hide, humiliated, my thoughts swarming.

Later, she apologizes and I forgive her, and after that, she never so much as raises her voice at me again. Still, I realize then that my family legacy of violent emotion did not skip my grandmother after all, and that she only learned to be very good at hiding what she inherited. Which means both that this legacy lives on in me and that I will have to learn to hide it as well.

MORE IMAGES: THE FACES OF Aunt Tina's friends. Charlene, who owns a beauty salon down the street and presses my hair every two weeks; Toni, a seamstress, who owns a store that sells fancy gowns she makes by hand; Melody, who has a collection of elegant purses and is the only person I know who makes me laugh more than Tina. These women witness my mother's tantrums and afterward look at me with worried expressions and assure me she loves me. I know that, I tell them. Of course she does. She has to. I'm her daughter.

Still more: the rolling green acres of Houston's wealthiest neighborhood, River Oaks, where, at seven, I'm enrolled in a K–12 private school as a scholarship student, and where I discover, to my absolute shock, that a whole other world has been, all this time, running smoothly alongside mine. The children at this school all live in matching mansions, go to the same summer camps, have parents who grew up rich together, share private jets, and use one another's beach houses interchangeably. St. John's will gain some notoriety in the late nineties for being the inspiration for and shooting location of *Rushmore*, Wes Anderson's cult classic prep school film, and even more in the 2010s as the alma mater of Elizabeth Holmes, the biotech billionaire whose business will turn out to have been built on fraud, but at the time it's known primarily as the best private school in the city.

My mother buys teacher's editions of every textbook, shows up at parent conferences ready to come to blows over my honor, drives to the school's vast and intimidating campus on her lunch break to deliver the finished homework I am forever leaving behind. In second grade, when I bring home a spelling test with ten points taken off for bad handwriting, she forces me to practice writing each week's exam words nightly and to start over if every letter isn't docked perfectly to the line beneath it.

But twice, she accidentally drops me off at school with a lunch bag packed with three green apples, two cans of pineapple, and nothing else. Once, she sends me with leftover beans from Frenchy's, the fried chicken stand where she'd picked up dinner the previous night, still in the same flimsy cardboard to-go container they came in. The cardboard melts open in the coatroom, making a mess, and a boy I have a crush on makes fun of me.

When I tell my mother this story, crying, she cannot stop laughing. She spends her days inserting catheters and cleaning bedpans and wiping up poor people's shit at a public hospital. To her, being liked by other students who attend a school like mine is entirely beside the point. Who cares if I impress them? What matters is that I impress her. And at least I have lunch and a dedicated parent who will pack it for me. She never had that. Her mother was always at work.

...

SOME BLACK PARENTS TELL THEIR children they have to work twice as hard to get half as far in a white-dominated society. When it comes to my mother, I do not need to be twice as good because of white people or society. I need to be twice as good for her.

When I spend a week at Girl Scout camp learning how to sail, she says we'll buy a boat so I can become a champion sailor. When I take a photography class at the Museum of Fine Arts, she says we'll turn the garage into a darkroom. When I find out a cousin is going to Berkeley and decide I want to go there too, she decides we'll pick up and move to California right away. But when I admit I don't actually want to move to a different state away from all my friends and our family, her face falls and she yells at me until I cry.

And, later, when I'm filling up the car on the way to school and I lose my grip and douse myself with gasoline, she drops me off anyway, my uniform skirt soaked through.

In first-period math, everyone around me whispers.

"What's that smell?" Ms. Sims finally asks.

"I spilled gasoline on myself," I say and shrug. Ms. Sims is everyone's favorite teacher, and one of the school's only Black instructors. She makes fun of me gently, laughs in a way that makes it so I'm in on the joke rather than its object. In doing so, she ensures that no one will feel sorry for me as she sends me out of the classroom to call my grandmother to pick me up so I can change.

IT BOTHERS MY MOTHER THAT I want to fit in, that I don't hate the school full of people who benefit directly from the inequality that plagues her own poverty-stricken patients. Because I don't hate it. In fact, I love it. I love the competition. I love the grades and rules and uniforms. I love how our teachers make clear to all of us, tacitly, that upward progress comes about only as the result of combat, that we must always be prepared to win.

"You're cynical," she says on the drive to campus, "like all those white girls at your school."

"You say that all the time, but it doesn't mean anything. White people and Black people aren't that different," I say.

In the drop-off line ahead of us, a girl climbs out of a brand-new Mercedes SUV in her uniform, smooth hair reflecting the light. Her name is Carter or Evan or Lainey or Allison (two *l*'s) or Alison (one *l*), and her family's last name is on a hospital wing or an office building or a street sign downtown. She waves at me and I wave back, faking a smile.

"We are different," my mother says, her voice full of its usual anger but also tinged with pity. "We are."

MY GRANDMOTHER BUYS US A house in an upscale section of Third Ward called Riverside Terrace. It's on Parkwood Drive, where Beyoncé Knowles and her sister, Solange, still live with their parents. The house has three bedrooms, stairs, hardwood floors, a backyard patio, and a detached garage with a laundry room in it. My mother, who resents my grandmother for this purchase, lets the house rot, covering the dining room table with laundry, leaving food on dishes in the kitchen sink for days.

When my grandmother hires a woman to clean, my mother locks her bedroom door and refuses to let her in. She tells me we're going to move to Atlanta, where she won't have to be bothered by my grandmother anymore, or Newark, where neither one of us will ever have to deal with white people ever again, or Africa, where she will figure out what part of the continent we are from so we can go back there. I like when she says "we." Like the idea of us figuring out where we came from together. Like the idea that I belong to her.

BUT I ALSO LIKE THIS other world I've stumbled into, where everything gleams. No one at St. John's has to tell me to stop calling my mother "Mama" and start saying "Mom." To say "parents" when I mean my grandmother, mother, and aunt. I only figure out gradually that doing so will help me better disguise myself among children bred for success.

"You're not poor," my friend Kevin, who is over to do homework, says as he wanders the big, light-filled rooms of the house my grandmother bought us. He is the son of two orthopedic surgeons, and his own house is actually multiple houses surrounding a pool on an estate in Memorial. "How come everyone thinks you're poor?"

See! I remember thinking, proudly, ridiculously. *I'm not any different from you.*

SOMEONE FINDS A STRAY DOG on the street and my grandmother gives him to us to keep in our large backyard. She buys us a second dog to keep the first one company. Shortly thereafter, my mother drives us to a breeder outside the city and we bring home a third puppy. She makes me promise not to tell my grandmother how much she paid for her. I sit in the back of my mother's truck with the puppy for a long time, both of us bewildered by our sudden presence in each other's lives.

The dogs belong to me. I lie out with them on our deck. I leave the doors open to let them run free from the yard into the house and back again. I bathe them every weekend in the laundry room sink and pull ticks out of their fur with my fingernails.

One night, we run out of dog food and I ask my mother if she'll pick some up on her way home. She refuses. I am always asking for something. I can never leave her alone. I'm getting on her god-damn nerves. After she leaves, in a rage of my own, I throw a can of insect spray at my bedroom window, breaking it. I write her a note of apology, leave it at the bottom of the stairs, and wait for her to get home. When she does, she reads the note, then drags me out of my room and tells me to put all three dogs in the car.

The dogs stick their heads through the window of her truck, the hard wind making them sneeze. She drives to a strip mall off the highway, parks, gets out, then opens the car door. The dogs jump out. She closes the door and pulls out of the lot. Later I will wish more than anything that I'd gotten out of the car too. But in that moment, I'm so scared I can't breathe. I can barely see. It's as if someone has reached into my head and switched off the light.

I watch the dogs through the side mirrors chasing the car, trying to catch up, pink tongues lolling. As we head back up the feeder road and she doesn't turn around and drive back, I feel myself fly out of my body, grow more and more distant from the sound of the tires against the road. Back home, she tells me to take off my pants, bends me over the bathtub, and beats me with a belt until I finally start to cry. I lie awake that night and listen to the silence.

The quietness that once filled our apartment appears to fill this new house permanently. Laundry falls off the dining room table onto the floor and stays there. Dirty plates abandoned in the sink sprout maggots, which wiggle whitely as I spray them down the drain. I only speak to her when I have to, and when I do, I'm cold and polite, like I am talking to someone at a bus stop.

My English teacher writes an email home saying I've been listless in class. The email goes to my grandmother's account—it's my grandmother's contact information we list in the school directory, since my mother changes our home phone number often—and I find it left open on the computer at her office. No one ever writes the teacher back, and no one mentions the email to me. But, soon after, my mother comes into my room holding an article cut out from the newspaper.

"You know I love you, right?" She reads from it. "Even when I'm angry? I care about you and I want you to be happy?"

"What?" I say.

She waves the cut-out article at me. "Granny said I have to do this with you. If I don't, then you're going to need therapy when you're older." She laughs when she says the word "therapy," as if the very idea is a joke. I start to cry and tell her to get out of my room. She tells me she knows I'm only pretending to be sad about the dogs, that I act normal around my friends, then mope around in front of her. It's time for me to stop, she says.

Maybe it's then that I realize we are in a war.

I learn through experimentation that if I don't cry when she hits me with a belt, she doesn't hit as hard or for as long. Then I learn that if instead of crying I sing—Janet Jackson or Mariah Carey or Shania Twain—softly while the leather makes contact with my skin, she will laugh and look a little spooked by the incongruity, but she won't hit me anymore.

I start emailing colleges in eighth grade so admissions officers will know me by name. I become an expert at applying for grants and scholarships and financial aid for summer programs that will look good on my applications. I play the flute in wind ensemble and go out for a sport every season. I get a job at a French bakery in Rice Village, a shopping center in the upscale neighborhood around Rice University, and learn to foam milk for cappuccinos to the strict standards of our exacting clientele. I volunteer at a camp for children with disabilities. I take every AP class I can get into.

When I learn my lab partner in honors biology, Charlotte, who transferred in from a different school and already speaks French fluently, plans to apply to a yearlong exchange program in France, I decide to apply too. When we both get in and move to Brittany to live with host families for all of eleventh grade, I learn the loneliness of far away is different from the loneliness at home. It's lighter and more romantic. It is the loneliness of waking up at 6:00 a.m. to catch a bus in the rain, of the smell of baking bread wafting over an empty town square, not the heavy silence of the house on Parkwood with my mother, who is always either seething or crying or too cloyingly happy or asleep. I understand what it's going to feel like when I am free. I'll finish at St. John's, then go far away to a very good college, and after that, I will only ever go back home for weekend visits to see my grandmother and Tina.

But the month before I'm supposed to leave France and return to the United States, my mother calls to ask if I want to transfer out of St. John's when I get back to Texas. Wouldn't I rather go to Lamar, the public high school next door? I'm devastated. I can't leave St. John's with its excellent Ivy League placement rates and thorough college advisory program. Attendance there is a crucial part of my plan to escape so I can have the life I want.

What appears to have happened was this: I took the SAT while I was abroad. I did well. So well that when my mother received my scores by mail, she called my ninth-grade Algebra II teacher, against whom she still held a grudge for complaining I stared out the window instead of paying attention in class. On the phone, my mother bragged about my score, told the teacher she was an asshole, and threatened her.

The problem goes away thanks to Mrs. Sims, who works in school administration now and has become a friend. After the school year starts, she calls me into her office under the pretense of discussing camera equipment for the yearbook, of which I am an editor. "Is your mom okay?" she asks.

"We don't know," I say, as if this is something "we" as a family have ever seriously discussed. It is not, the consensus simply that my mother cannot handle a lot of stress.

Mrs. Sims changes the subject back to the yearbook, and I know she's trying to spare my feelings, but I want to keep talking about it. I'm seventeen and no one has ever asked me this question before.

...

32

SENIOR YEAR, I WIN A National Scholastic Gold Key award for a short story I write called "The Pigeon God," about two little boys who kill an old man who lives in a park. My mother comes with me to the local awards ceremony at a convention room in a hotel downtown. So does my best friend, Amy. When the woman running the event calls my name, I walk to the front of the room to stand next to her for a photograph. She hands me a gold pin and a copy of *Housekeeping* by Marilynne Robinson.

"Are your parents here? They must be so proud of you," the woman says.

"Here I am," my mother says from the audience in her tiny voice, lightly touched with a Southern twang. She stands up in the back of the room. "That's my baby." The crowd titters. She looks so small and so vulnerable and so proud. At the end of the night, when I tell her I'm going out to dinner with Amy and she hugs me goodbye, Amy gawks at us and says to me later, "You two hug like you've never even met." I realize she's right, and I think, *Good. Let the world consider us strangers.*

AMY AND I GO TO neighboring colleges in Providence, Rhode Island. Our first month, she almost gets us both arrested for walking around with bolt cutters in the middle of the night, spray-painting our names on a parking lot wall. I beg the cops not to take us in while she glares at them, blasé. "You're the smart one, I guess," they say to me before they let us go. And it's true, I am, but I have to be so I can take care of her.

In high school, every boy we know is desperately and unabashedly in love with Amy. For the rest of my life, she will always be the marker by which I measure every other girl. Her beauty and charisma make us popular, get us invited to parties thrown by upperclassmen and free tickets to concerts when the indie bands we like pass through town. We come home from these concerts in the early hours of the morning, hair heavy with the smell of smoke and beer, backstage-access wristbands hanging from our skinny arms. As soon as we get to Providence, she falls for a boy who shortly thereafter drops out of RISD to ride trains across the country. Meanwhile, I date an organic chemistry major from Beverly Hills. Amy describes him as "clean" though really she means "rich."

You certainly have a fetish for white guys, she messages me after she meets him for the first time. Her mother is Chinese and her father is from Singapore.

Maybe white guys have a fetish for me, I message her back. But she isn't wrong. Whiteness seems to me then to mean money. Money means safety. Safety means control. Control means a comfortable sense that today won't be all that different from the next.

But, after spending our entire lives in Texas, Amy and I both find ourselves stunned by the bleakness of Providence in winter. By sophomore year, it becomes clear that neither one of us will find our footing in this place. Amy, after ending things with her boyfriend and breaking out in boils that leave pits in her perfect face, transfers to school in Austin, and even though everything in me wants to leave with her, I stay.

THREE

I MEET SADIE, THE GIRL who becomes my best friend at Brown, at an orientation program for Black students. We grow close over a love of Goldschläger and a common enemy in the other girls studying literature, with their shiny hair, and eating disorders that make them look frail and breakable, like little, brittle Joan Didions in training. These girls write about their beauty, their vulnerability, the sadness that mars their sun-dappled lives, in a way that makes their future literary success seem assured. "They shrug this place off like they don't even need it, but I need it," I say to Sadie.

"Then take it," she answers. "Why not? You're here."

To Sadie, information is useful or it is not, people are worth thinking about or they are not, certain conversations are worth her time or they are not. She's the type of person America was built for, and it seems to me that she will thrive, no matter what. She isn't like me, in that she fits squarely at the center of the Brown population while I hover somewhere in its orbit, feeling as if I'm always meant to be expressing my gratitude. We both know this and recognize our relative positions, and that recognition, whether we want it to or not, informs everything we say and do in each other's presence.

SADIE'S BIRTHDAY PARTY, WHICH SHE throws every year, is an annual campus event, and each year it grows larger and lasts longer, peopled with rich legacy admits, the children of celebrities and business tycoons, drawn in by our collective heat. One year, before her party, we go to the Providence Place mall for outfits and come back with matching shoes, hers pink and mine gold. In my memory we picked them out individually, but later I'll overhear her telling our friends that I saw her pick out the shoes and then asked for the same ones in a different color. It's entirely possible that this is true. After that same party, I take the organic chemistry major back to my dorm room and have sex for the first time, having planned it so I will always remember the date.

On a different night, Sadie hands me a page to read, a meditation she wrote for her poetry class about a woman taking a train home from a night out. It's gorgeous, in a way I know my own work is not. "My professor said she wishes she could write like this," she tells me. She isn't boasting. She sounds perplexed. She came to college to be a doctor and signed up for Poetry I on a whim, and now look. It's like this for her. Life falls into place.

THE ORGANIC CHEMISTRY MAJOR INTRODUCES me to sushi at a restaurant that sits forgotten in the corner of a mini-mall halfway between campus and town. On weekends we drive to Newport to look at the old houses built into the cliffs, to Boston to visit his friends at Harvard, to Pawtucket to watch the leaves turn. We spend afternoons at the campus library reading upstairs in the dark, sharing a carrel. He invites me home to spend spring break with him at his parents' house in a gated community off Mulholland Drive, and when his mom and dad come to find us in baggage claim at LAX, his mother looks directly through me, as if she's looking for a girlfriend who is white.

"I'm Sarah!" I say brightly, ignoring her shock. I shake her hand.

We drive to Zuma Beach, where he goes surfing with people he knew in high school. I watch from the sand with the other girlfriends, who all went to the same L.A. private school and don't understand why I am there. We go on a long walk through the nature reserve that butts up against his backyard. At night when his parents are out, we dress up and have pasta and wine at the dining table. He lights a tapered candle and smiles at me through its flame. I imagine us older and living in a house like this one, our hair going gray and every day the same. I start to cry.

"It feels too much like we're my parents, huh?" he says, picking up our plates to take them to the sink. "It's freaking you out." And he's right. It's too much. We have both said we love each other, but it's occurring to me now that I don't know how, and maybe don't want, to be loved.

THE CULTURE AT BROWN UNIVERSITY demands that all students at least want to make the world a better place, and I do want this, yes, but I also want to ensure I will never have to go back home, which means I will have to figure out how to become rich. I'm not good enough at lab work to be pre-med and I can't figure out how exactly one signs up to be pre-law. I channel my anxiety into shoveling bagels into my mouth then throwing them up in a secret bathroom under the cafeteria stairs. I write down everything I eat with the calorie count next to it. It's exhausting, this project, but gratifying to the part of my brain dedicated to keeping score.

I take fiber pills and text Sadie: How much weight do you think it's possible to lose from a poop?

She texts me back: This has got to stop.

"What do you have to be depressed about?" my mother asks when I call home. "Nothing."

"Okay, then. I won't be depressed anymore," I say and start to cry.

"I've worked too hard for you," she says. "And whatever it is that's wrong now, I will not let you blame me for it."

What do I have to be depressed about? I don't know. I think it's the fact that it never stops snowing in Providence. When it isn't snowing it's raining, the campus sitting dead under a layer of ice.

I call my grandmother and say, "I feel as if I'm attached to a rope floating farther and farther away. I can see the earth, but I can't get to it. Have you ever felt like that? What did you do?"

"Well," she says, "I had two children."

This is not an option for me at this time. I do, through a friend with connections to a pharmacist in Boston, have access to an unlimited supply of Dexedrine. The campus doctor knows nothing of this and so prescribes me birth control for mood regulation. Unaware of the dangers of mixing both medications with copious amounts of alcohol, I remain under the impression that the Rhode Island winter is the reason I want to die.

The organic chemistry major and I go to his ski house in Mammoth. I take a hallucinogen for the first time and refuse to let him touch me. We move in together anyway the following semester, and something about the unwashed dishes in our kitchen keeps sending me into rages. One morning, I find myself pulling plates off the counter and dropping them on the floor.

"Dirty dishes really get to you, babe," he says, wrapping his arms around my shoulders and guiding me into his chest.

I cheat on him with boys who smoke a lot of weed and who don't like me very much. They hurt my feelings, and I go back to him and for some reason he lets me. One night, though, I bring one of these boys home to our apartment while he is there. "You respect nothing," he says to me, angrier than I've ever seen anyone other than my mother. His anger takes me by surprise, and even he seems thrown off balance by it.

SADIE FALLS FOR A BOY in our friend group, a tall, dreadlocked artist who likes all the same music she does, and they disappear into each other. Feeling abandoned and no longer really able to go back to the apartment I share with my boyfriend, I shift into a different circle made up of white kids from high-cost-of-living cities who communicate in obscure one-liners and do bad coke and drink cheap beer. I want upward social mobility. They're in the process of pissing away decades of generational wealth. My hope is we can meet in the middle.

So when I'm invited to go with the group into Manhattan to spend the weekend at someone's parents' empty penthouse, I say yes. Two slingback chairs in the living room are, we are told, made of reindeer skin, which suggests to my brain something illicit. The heated bathroom floors and the reindeer-skin chairs and the apartment's location on the Upper East Side seem to me the height of luxury and strangeness and I feel proud of myself for being there, as if I have accomplished something important.

So I drink and do drugs and it's possible the boy whose apartment it is and I cut one another with razor blades naked in a bathtub to see the blood. We aren't attracted to each other. I've slept with one or two of his friends, but he and I don't have that kind of rapport, and as far as I know he isn't straight. Nevertheless, we fall asleep in his bed and a few minutes or maybe an hour later, I wake up to feel his penis thrusting into me as rough and hard as stone.

Maybe, I remember thinking, he's having sex with me while I am asleep ironically? Maybe it's my fault for not getting the joke? These boys never say or do anything in earnest. Their detachment is why other people find them compelling. I elbow him backward and whisper in a voice like my mother at her most furious: *stop it*. And he stops, rolls over onto his back, laughs, a little embarrassed, and falls asleep again. I do too. Only when I wake up does it occur to me something wrong has happened, something more wrong than I expected or planned for.

Back on campus, I feel worse than ever before. It's as if the whole fallen industrial city is colluding in making me feel terrible, with its burned-out, abandoned warehouses and piles of black snow. The organic chemistry major and I still have each other's email passwords, and I log in to his to find a message from his sister. "It's not her fault, but she's not a good person," she writes. She is begging him to please move on from me.

Whose fault is it, then? I wonder. How can it not be my fault what kind of person I am? I develop a habit of gouging away at my body, leaving ridges in my thighs with whatever sharp edge I can find.

IN HOUSTON FOR SPRING BREAK my senior year, I go out to a bar with Amy and our high school friends. The organic chemistry major and I have broken up definitively, and he is dating someone else. I don't want to have to move back in with my mother, but to stop this from happening I have to graduate from college, and I don't want to go back to Providence. All my friends have jobs lined up, but when I look to the future I see a wall. At the bar, I get too drunk and yell at everyone. On the way home, Amy is in awe. "It was like you were possessed," she says. "You were so angry."

In the car with my mother on my way to the airport the next morning, I, once again, cannot stop crying. She threatens to take me to the Harris County Psychiatric Center, where the doctors will put me in a straitjacket and force pills down my throat. The hospital is down the road from our old house on Parkwood Drive in Riverside Terrace. She made this same threat often when I was a child, but what neither of us knows then is that this is the same hospital she will end up in a decade from now.

Meanwhile, I get out of the car at a stoplight. I walk until I find a payphone, then call Aunt Tina to pick me up. I have missed my flight and I decide I will take this as a sign that I do not have to go back to Brown. Back home, though, my grandmother tells me calmly that I cannot stay in Houston, that I have to return to school, and that if I don't, I'll have ruined my life.

My grandmother's advice tends, in general, toward the gnomic: she quotes Thoreau; tells me to know myself; tells me life, unexamined, is not worth living. This is the first and only time she will tell me concretely what I need to do. And I do it because she is right.

SADIE IS THE FIRST PERSON who, when I tell her about my mother, says, I didn't know. I had no idea. I'm so sorry. How you were treated wasn't normal. It matters that it happened and you're not wrong to think it does.

"Have you ever thought about going on antidepressants?" she continues. I'm back in Providence and we are sitting in the living room of my apartment, which is shrouded in absolute darkness even though it is only 4:30.

"Do you have any idea how bad those are for your liver?" I say.

"So your plan is to kill yourself without damaging your liver?" Sadie says.

I haven't gone outside in days and I still cannot stop crying. My grades are in shambles. I've flaked on multiple group projects and my professors keep emailing me to find out where I am. And it's true that I've been thinking about the Tylenol PM at the nearby twenty-four-hour convenience store and wondering how much I would have to take to not wake up again.

"What about a therapist?" Sadie says.

But the idea of talking at length about my mother terrifies me—I feel certain she will hear me, fly to campus, and drag me out of any psychologist's office by my chin. Her fingernails will leave moon-shaped wounds in my face that, later, I will deepen with my own.

But Sadie will not leave me alone until I promise to do *something*. The therapist I do finally agree to see gives me books with pastel covers titled *Anorexia* and *Bulimia*. "Would you like to take these home?" she asks. No, I say. I would not. A second therapist, who is Black, tells me I have too many white friends and suggests I start going to parties thrown by Black students, try to date more Black men. It is a solution that appeals to me, though the options in both areas at Brown are slim. After three sessions, she tells me she can't see me anymore—university rules—and suggests a third therapist in the city who turns out not to take my insurance.

AFTER GRADUATION I GET AN assistant job through a friend at an entertainment agency in Beverly Hills. But on the day I'm supposed to start, I cannot bring myself to leave the guest room of the family friend's house where I am staying in Los Angeles. I call my mother, crying, and she asks me if I'm on drugs and then suggests I'm going to die in a dumpster with a syringe stuck in my ass like Anna Nicole Smith. It is true that Anna Nicole Smith died recently of a drug overdose, though not exactly in this way. Nevertheless, she manages to work herself up into such a lather at the idea that I would do this to her—that I would *die*—after all she's done for me, that we both have to get off the phone. I call Aunt Tina, who listens to me cry for a while, then tells me to forget the job and come back to Houston.

I stay in my grandmother's condo for a month, sleeping on her couch. My mother is no longer taking my calls, but I have dreams in which we are shouting at each other while the city falls down all around us and the car we are in breaks into pieces. I wake up struggling to breathe.

A therapist I see in Houston courtesy of my grandmother, who offers to pay the bill, has big hair and a deep southern drawl and a large, comforting bosom. I tell her all about the organic chemistry major, whose new girlfriend's father runs a movie studio in Los Angeles. She is more interested in talking about the absence of my own father. "Do you realize how afraid of men you are?" she says. I had not. I apply for an administrative job at the University of Houston to get health insurance to pay for more therapy.

When I get a phone call asking me to come in for an interview, I go to Aunt Tina's friend Charlene to get my eyebrows waxed. Each time she touches me, I flinch. I notice her notice my flinching. She loves my family, she says as she layers wax above my eyelids, but I don't need to stay here. Go to California, she says. I know you think because your grandmother and your mother and your Aunt Tina all stayed here, you have to, too. But you don't. Everybody doesn't live this way.

I CANCEL THE INTERVIEW AND apply for a job as an assistant at a different entertainment agency in Los Angeles. I move into an apartment in Koreatown with two people I know from college and immediately start sleeping with one of them while casually alien-ating the other. I use my new health insurance to see Linda, a ther-apist who appears to openly hate me. My real problem, she says, is that I've never seen anybody work hard. "No one understands me," she says, repeating my complaints back to me in a voice pitched up to resemble my own. "Don't be so dramatic," she commands. The economy, post-2008 housing collapse, is in free fall, and she does not have time for my bullshit. I keep seeing her every two weeks anyway, because she charges me a sliding-scale rate and because in spite of the way she talks to me, I sometimes feel as if she is my only real friend in the city.

It's Sadie who, applying for MFA programs in creative writing while she works as a community organizer in Detroit, sends me her guidebooks so I can apply, too. You have to be relentless, she tells me. We send each other our personal statements and she shares with me the spreadsheets she's made with every application's due dates clearly marked so that we can hold each other accountable.

IN SERVICE OF THIS NEW goal, I sign up to take fiction classes at UCLA Extension. I join a writing group that meets weekly in an apartment downtown. I also go on a date with a filmmaker named Ethan whom I meet at a birthday party thrown for a friend at the agency where I'm an assistant.

When Ethan comes to pick me up the first time, I see his eyes light, a little judgmentally, on a line of coke laid out on the living room table by one of my roommates who got drunk and forgot to clean it up the night before. He looks horrified by my bedroom, so cluttered with clothes and bags and shoes the floor is barely visible, and even more so by our bathroom, about which the less said, the better. He invites me to his own quiet apartment down the street, which is immaculately clean, his bookshelf arranged alphabetically by genre, his pens divided by color, his computer keyboard, unlike mine, free of crumbs. He's got no roommates, is five years older than me, and seems to be the first true grown-up I've met in L.A.

The name for what Ethan is isn't "ambitious," because ambition requires acknowledging an alternative to getting what you want, which is not a possibility he appears to have considered. He is about to leave Los Angeles to direct his first feature in suburban Boston using money he raised himself after partnering with producers he met at film festivals where his graduate school thesis film played. Coincidentally, his leaving coincides with the month my lease will end and my roommates plan to give up the house we share. He offers me his empty apartment for the two months he'll be gone while I look for a new one.

We spend a hot summer afternoon carrying IKEA furniture out of my place and into his while sweat pours down the back of his neck and stains his T-shirt. He unloads my things onto the carpet and says to me, sounding a little resigned, "No food in here. Okay? No eating on the couch. No putting cups down without coasters. No spilling." I make a joke about hosting an orgy in his bedroom. He doesn't laugh, and then he's gone, leaving me to poke through his closet full of old *New Yorker*s organized by date, his box sets of Ingmar Bergman films, his Tarkovsky Blu-rays.

In an effort to understand him better, I watch his favorite

movie, *Stalker*, from 1979, shot on grainy celluloid in sepia tones. It's about three men on a journey to a secret room that holds their hearts' desires, and although almost nothing seems to actually happen in it, in each individual shot, I can sense a rumbling core.

WHEN I AM NOT AT work or at home watching Ethan's movies, I am putting together my application to NYU's MFA program, applying with the stories I wrote in my UCLA Extension class. I submit my application with a jargon-laden personal statement about Toni Morrison and Aristotle's *Poetics* and William Faulkner, trying to incorporate everything I learned in college that might sound impressive. I don't get in.

"Maybe I'm not good enough," I say to Ethan.

"Why would you say that?" he asks. The question isn't rhetorical. He wants to know. What purpose could such a thought ever serve?

I apply to NYU again, this time with new stories and a personal statement about a fiction workshop I took with the novelist John Edgar Wideman, who once told us, exasperated because no one had done the reading for that day, that we needed to find the thing we wanted to structure our lives around. I write honestly that I believe I've found that thing. This time, to my complete surprise, I'm accepted. The school offers full tuition remission and a stipend to live on for the two years I'm there.

Meanwhile, Ethan finds us a one-bedroom apartment in Los Feliz. It's on my favorite street in the city, and, even better, it is rent-controlled, which means that, as long as we live there, we will both always be able to afford to write. We move in together, our books mingled on our shelves, my dresses in the hallway closet hanging in between his coats. It's a gift he's found for us, this place, and in exchange, I promise that when school is over I will come back.

THE SUMMER BEFORE I LEAVE for New York, my favorite cousin on my father's side gets married. Ethan and I take the Coast Starlight train from Los Angeles to Sonoma Valley and meet up with my dad's large Catholic family on a golf course decorated with white flowers. After the ceremony we eat Mediterranean appetizers on the deck of a country club. My dad, a very tall man with yellow-brown skin and freckles, comes over to say what he always says when he sees me, which is that he wants to buy acres of land and build a chalet and give all his kids keys so they can come by anytime they want. Do some writing. Play some music. A quiet cottage where we can all pop through.

My dad, who currently lives at his mom's house in Oakland, has eight children by four different women, some of whom are at the wedding. His other exes—who, like my mother are short, medium brown, and bird-boned—still flirt with him when they see him and appear to indulge him like a sweet younger brother. Something about my dad makes women want to take care of him. Women aside from my mother and me, that is. For my part, I can't bring myself to listen to or return the long voicemails he leaves me every year on my birthday telling me he loves me because I never know how to respond. Now I dance away from him as he talks, knowing if I stay for too long he will start to brag about his championship-winning high school basketball team or about a pet theory of his that he can trace our lineage to Sitting Bull.

Afterward, my father's sister Paula drives us back to the hotel. A lawyer in Sacramento, she is thin and put-together, with salt-and-pepper hair, long, tapered fingers, and a nose the exact same shape and size as mine. I tell her what my dad said about the chalet, laughing, expecting her to laugh too—he is the black sheep of his siblings, and the only one who still lives at home. Instead she looks sad. "There's a lot about your dad you probably don't know," she says.

She tells me their father—my grandfather—worked for TWA as a mechanic and lost his job shortly before his second-youngest son, my dad's older brother, began to die of multiple sclerosis. My dad was the youngest of eight, the only child home to watch his brother deteriorate. As we reach the hotel, she tells me to call her later so she can tell me more.

"Okay," I say again, but never do. I don't want to hear any more sad stories about my family history. I'm happy that summer, but I can still feel dread layered under the happiness like hot tar. I'm not in the mood to map my father's tragic backstory out so far that it meets my mother's and I can start to see the beginnings of my own.

IN THE MORNING, I WAKE up to a wall of emails from my mother, new ones appearing as she sends them to me in manic sprints. The messages read like curses. They exhale a special kind of heat that makes me want to run somewhere secret, somewhere no one can touch me. She's enraged because last time we talked, I mentioned

I'm taking antibiotics prescribed for mild, persistent acne. She sends diagrams of failing hearts and sclerotic kidneys and damaged nervous systems. She tells me I'll wind up in a hospital bed hooked up to machines. I'll overtax my nervous system and it will never snap back. Stroke. Heart attack. All the terrible diseases she has watched her elderly patients die of will come now for me.

"What is it?" Ethan asks, emerging from the bathroom. He's been changing for a hike and finds me sitting in the corner on the floor.

I snap at him. "It's nothing. Leave me alone."

"Stop being mean to me," he says. He's calm, matter-of-fact.

I shut my laptop and hold it up against my chest like a shield. I used to think everyone screamed terrible things when they got angry, never apologized, then went on as if nothing had happened at all. I'm learning from Ethan this isn't true. Perhaps because he grew up in a house run by psychology professors, he falls into a therapeutic mood when I'm angry, responding to my emotions rather than the insults I fling at his head. I'm still trying to learn, from him, how to operate in these situations.

"It's just," I say, "my mom is so fucked and my dad is so fucked, it's impossible for me to imagine a life for myself that isn't also fucked."

"If you think you can predict the future, you're crazy," Ethan says. "Your mother and father both happen to have extremely bad luck."

Not long before this wedding, I'd gone home with Ethan to his parents' house in Boston for the first time. The day we arrived, his mother invited me out on an errand and I froze, mute with terror. We drove to a garden supply store, where she picked out a gift for a friend. She pointed out sheep in a field by the side of the road. She asked if I wanted to go with her to an aerobics class the next day. This was what it had always been like for Ethan, I realized. Not once had his mother shoved his head against the closed car window while he rode quietly in the passenger seat, or grabbed his arm so hard it bled, or ranted at him unrelentingly for miles on the highway for reasons he didn't understand. It was simply not the type of thing it would cross her mind to do.

Part of me suspects sometimes my mother was right about what she said in the school drop-off line when I was a kid. Ethan and I are so different, the possibility of a life like my mother's so unimaginable to him, I may as well be talking to him in a language he doesn't speak. It is astonishing to me that he or anyone could so easily file both of my parents' lives under the rubric of "bad luck."

IN NEW YORK THAT FALL, I am struck by a curiously incapacitating digestive illness that causes food to sit inside my stomach for what feels like days, slicing up my intestines as it breaks down. Blessed with decent health insurance through my graduate fellowship, I get CT scans and an MRI. Every specialist sends me to someone new. I travel back and forth from the health services office to NYU Langone. I pass each moment I'm not in class or at the doctor in shock from discomfort, struggling to breathe through the pain.

A neurologist at NYU has me push against her hands with all my strength, a test of my nervous system, then diagnoses me with anxiety. I speak calmly, professionally, with all the private school in my voice I can muster: I'm in graduate school for creative writing. I've come here on a full fellowship. Because for a brief period I don't have to worry about money, I am actually less stressed than I have been for a long time. And while I understand stress can cause symptoms like the ones I'm describing, what if the reason behind them is something else? Something medical that she can help me fix? But this is not a possibility the neurologist seems willing to entertain. And after appointments like this at clinics and hospitals across the city, I soon grow too tired to argue.

Desperate, I find a therapist who focuses on healing illness through the body. Her name is Anne. I tell her the truth, that I am afraid my mom will know that I am in therapy and she will be angry with me. It's 2011, and my mother and I are speaking again after a long period of her shutting me out for my having chosen to take prescription medication. As if I've been adequately punished for this crime through my illness, she's answering my calls again. She emails me YouTube clips of songs she listened to when I was a baby: Otis Redding, Al Green, Sam Cooke. She is also investigating her father's untimely death—the mysterious suicide that may have been a murder—and has sent me his autopsy report. We talk on the phone about him every other day. This is the longest we've gone without fighting in ages, and the thought of her going back to not speaking to me makes me want to curl up into a ball.

Anne holds her hands out to me, palms touching. She wants me to try an exercise. To imagine I am in one of her hands and my mother is in the other. Slowly she spreads her hands apart.

"How does that feel?" she asks.

Like an ache in my chest. A longing in the oldest part of me without words.

She suggests auditory eye movement desensitization and reprocessing therapy (EMDR), a therapeutic method designed for people with PTSD. At our first session, she hands me a pair of headphones. I put them on and hear a beep, first in one ear, then the other. She asks me questions about the past while the beeps play. The movement in combination with the sound is supposed to erase the negative emotions associated with certain memories. We start with small irritations—an old man eating a messy sandwich in the park who once commanded me to smile—and work our way up to greater traumas. After three sessions, I tell her about the dogs, my mother dropping them off in the parking lot, their faces in the side-view mirror. The room dissolves. I'm in the passenger seat of my mom's white truck, watching the dogs run after us, and I can't breathe.

"What color is the wall?" Anne asks.

I describe the painting above her desk, an anodyne vase filled with purple flowers on a table and then I am back in the present, seated on her sofa.

"You're okay. You're okay. You're okay," she says. She tells me to gently stroke my own arm with the opposite hand and repeat this phrase until I feel better. This is a coping mechanism I can use in the future whenever things hurt too much.

I tell Anne the EMDR therapy worked, because she seemed convinced it would. Encouraged, she suggests yoga, meditation, and deep breathing, and I sign up for all the classes she suggests but don't go.

SADIE IS ALSO IN GRADUATE school in New York. Her mentor, a poet who won the National Book Award, invites her to drinks with a different poet who won a Pulitzer. Sadie asks me to come as her guest. No matter how far ahead of me she gets, she is always reaching a hand back, trying to pull me up to where she is.

It's starting to feel like a drag, following Sadie around. So this time I say no. On the phone, Ethan tells me he doesn't understand why I left L.A. if I'm not going to go to bars with Pulitzer Prize–winning poets when invited. If, instead, I'm going to sit in my bedroom and be sad.

"I hate to say it, but you're in New York City on a creative writing fellowship. It doesn't exactly get better than this."

"What would you know? You're a fundamentally happy person."

"You went there for a reason," Ethan says. "If you don't start putting yourself in the mindset that this is going to eventually work out, it won't."

"Sure," I say. "It's just—"

"No. It's not just anything."

The problem with depression is that, like alcoholism, it's an illness people get annoyed at you for having. ("Everybody's depressed," Linda, my old therapist, once said to me, as if the cure lay in integrating this singular fact once and for all into my worldview.)

When Sadie gets an internship in the poetry department at *The New Yorker*, she invites me to drop her name so I can land an internship in the fiction department. It works, and, once a week for the next year, I take the train to Midtown so I can read the slush pile, short stories submitted by people who hope their writing might someday appear in the magazine's illustrious font. Much of what I come across is exceptional, but almost no one will ever know this, because almost no one will ever look at it, even if it does somehow magically find its way into print somewhere. I like how it seems as if everyone—from the writers to the editors—understands obscurity to be a condition of the field; how, as a result, the stakes feel both low and intimidatingly high. I submit my own writing to the literary journals that pile up in my cubicle, free copies a perk of the job, and rack up a pile of rejections. My time at the magazine becomes the only time when I feel as if I am inside the world and not floating somewhere near it or above it.

Sadie publishes a poem in a well-regarded online journal and says she is sure if I submit, they'll take one of my stories, too. I send in a story about a girl who leaves her corporate job and starts a business selling fruit, then steals a baby from her neighbor, and they accept it. Then, Sadie works her way onto the masthead of a political review. Right away, she commissions me to write a piece about state-sanctioned violence. In my piece, I include a sentence about certain moments that "stop you in your tracks and force you to react. That force you to stop thinking about your life as a movie, and start thinking about your life as your life."

You can't generalize a sentiment like that, Sadie notes in the margins in her edits. *Not everybody feels this way.*

Sadie doesn't. Her life is her life. Not something she witnesses, but something she does. I want to be like that, but I'm not. And so, I stand beside her and I watch.

FOUR

THE ARCADES PROJECT WASN'T A book written to be read for pleasure. It wasn't written to be read at all. In a letter to a friend composed deep into its undertaking, Benjamin wrote that "not a syllable" of the work he planned to create existed yet.[7] Today it reads like an extremely long and detailed blueprint for something more complete, the manuscript comprising hundreds of pages of images and notes and paragraphs pulled from other texts. The work Benjamin planned to organize out of them was interrupted first by his flight from Vichy France into Spain in 1940 and then by his suicide.

When I finally read the entire thousand-page volume in the summer of 2012, I enter what feels like a fugue state. I'm in Paris at the time, working as a residential advisor for NYU's undergraduate creative writing program. The book's strange juxtapositions color everything I see, so that even as I'm making dinner reservations and requesting photocopies and helping the students board the metro, I feel always on the verge of epiphany, as if I'm always just about to understand the universe.

Take, for example, the tree growing through the window of the fourth-floor room in the student residence where I live. It occurs to me, looking at it one day, that its branches mirror the veins in my arm. Watching a documentary about the limestone caverns under Paris, I notice their shape mirrors the city's branching network of streets and the patterns on broken squares of sidewalk. Crossing a bridge, I look down at the river rushing beneath me and think, at the same time, of the subway tunnels and catacombs that divide the city's foundations. Everything flying apart as it holds together. All of us alive at the same time as we are dying. It's as if I've discovered some unspoken truth no one ever bothered to share with me: stare at anything long enough and you'll start to see it crack.

My old honors biology lab partner, Charlotte, now pursuing a PhD in comparative literature, comes to Paris for a conference. We walk in the rain to the Jewish quarter while I tell her about the heat I feel building up behind my eyes, about the correlations between plants and streets and veins and rivers that appear to point to a unifying factor I can see but not quite explain. She suggests a book, a collection of Benjamin's essays called *Illuminations*. Reading it, I come across this line in the introduction by Hannah Arendt: "He was concerned with the correlation between a street scene, a speculation on the stock exchange, a poem, a thought, with the hidden line which holds them together."[8]

THAT NIGHT, I SEARCH BENJAMIN'S name on Wikipedia. The results come back in French, so I open another window and draw up the same entry in English, noting the differences between the two: Wikipedia informs me that Benjamin's wealthy father invested in German ice-skating rinks, while French Wikipedia—Wikipédia—does not. Wikipédia makes no mention of Benjamin's health as a child, while Wikipedia reads good-naturedly, "Personally, he was a boy of fragile health." Both entries describe his father as a banker, but only Wikipédia specifies that Benjamin lived primarily on inherited money. Wikipédia makes it clear that Benjamin killed himself after learning, falsely, that he would be sent back to Vichy France from Spain, where he was attempting to flee to the United States. Wikipedia informs the reader that he killed himself, but not that the information that led him to do so was false. On Wikipédia, the subtitle for the section detailing his death is "Une Mort Tragique," while in English, it is simply "Death."

The entries suggest a universe that branches like the tree outside my window, like the veins in my arm, a set of parallel planes in which the same man led two different lives or, potentially, as many lives as internet encyclopedia entries about him in different languages exist.

MOST OF THE PARIS ARCADES were constructed in the early to mid-nineteenth century, and by the time Benjamin started writing about them almost a hundred years later, they had largely fallen into disrepair. A handful have been refurbished. I visit the Passage Jouffroy, a covered outdoor corridor in central Paris, and walk across the tile past art galleries, antiquarian bookstores, cafés, jewelers, and movie poster shops. Light shines dull and waxy through the glass roof, so that the items on all the shelves look like props in a play. In *The Arcades Project*, Benjamin describes the passageways' original faded light—gas lamps through glass ceilings—as a means of illuminating the past as it exists now, today, in the present. I imagine two businessmen I pass as red-faced peasants. I imagine their skinny waitress as a tubercular queen.

I use my NYU student ID to get into the Bibliothèque Nationale's reading room, where Benjamin himself spent years gathering research. At a long wooden table, I sketch out a story about a fictional French philosopher inspired by Benjamin named Nicholas Canton, who discovers the world is constantly breaking open, his own life in Paris one in an invisible many, like a leaf on a tree, each instant opening up forever and outward, blossoming into many.

Canton believes fate and destiny in each world are manifestations of this pattern of growth, which means the future might be easily calculable if one can only find a moment's exact origin point. He calls this tree-like growth pattern that governs the universe the Simultaneity and writes a book about it called *The Anatomy Book*, early chapters of which include a promise that Canton will provide the underlying equations necessary for travel through time. During the French Revolution, he is imprisoned and executed, and his work is destroyed by the Communards. However, some complete copies of the manuscript are rumored to have survived.

Over the next few days, the sketch turns into a novel that moves back and forth in time between Revolutionary-era Paris and present-day New England, where a graduate student named Mark is researching Canton with the help of Laura, his undergraduate assistant. As they search for a complete copy of Canton's manuscript with the equations intact, they also start sleeping together. In alternating chapters, the book follows Laura as an adult in New York. She's looking now for Mark, who abandoned her long ago in the middle of their research project. By the end of the book, the reader discovers the Laura in the future is not the same person as the Laura in college, but a different version of her in a different version of the world with Canton's science behind it. Soon I'm trapped in a morass of plot complicated, mostly, by Mark, the graduate student character, who, no matter how hard I try, I cannot make appealing or realistic. But still, I wake up every morning and write, first for days, then months, eventually for years, and feel all the different people I pretend to be merging into one.

I MOVE BACK TO LOS Angeles in 2013 and get a job in a university advancement office customizing form letters for large donors. The job supports my work on the novel—I have a cubicle with a printer in it and unlimited paper—but the task itself is so mind-numbingly dull that the misery it inspires makes me feel like I'm being lowered inch by inch into a pit. On the building's sixth floor is an entire department outfitted with wellness meditation CDs and biofeedback machines, the university having organized things so that we can address our depression without ever having to go outside. I make an appointment for a biofeedback session, and in it, I cry wordlessly.

An administrator tells me to think of my emotions as a river I can step in, even cross, without being carried away. Your emotions are not you, she explains. She gives me a set of recorded meditations on which a Santa Monica psychologist named Dr. Stephen Sideroff intones affirmations that suggest I create the world in my brain, that everything I feel stems from me, that if I can convince myself that I live a life full of positivity and abundance, then this will be my reality. *Dear Mr. and Mrs. Singh*, I tap out on my computer. *Thank you very much for your generosity to our athletics program. We deeply appreciate your strong support.*

You are the only person who can make yourself happy, urges Dr. Sideroff in my earbuds. *You must imagine leading the life that makes you happy.*

Sadie calls to tell me she sold her first poetry collection to a major publisher. I'm proud of her. I know how hard she worked. But I'm sad for me. So sad I want to draw a line down my wrist with a letter opener and step out of my skin, let the river of emotions carry me away. Sadie is going to move ahead without me and then I will lose her. I will work this terrible job forever and I will die here at my desk having accomplished nothing of note.

I turn off Dr. Sideroff's affirmations, get up from my desk, and walk out of the building onto Wilshire Boulevard. Behind the Westwood Branch Library is a cemetery where celebrities are buried. Marilyn Monroe, Hugh Hefner, Rodney Dangerfield. It's a place I like to go for a kind of dark reassurance. Death, in the end, will come for us all.

"Why can't I write faster?" I ask Ethan that night at home.

"Why don't you think you can write faster?" he replies. Then: "What the hell is wrong with you?"

I have dropped a coffee mug on the floor on purpose to watch it shatter.

"I feel like I'm dying. I think my job is trying to kill me. It's not a job for humans. It's not a job I can do and stay alive."

ETHAN TAKES ME ON A date to an event he read about on a flyer posted in the bathroom at Brū, the coffee shop across the street from our apartment. The event takes place at the Lyric Hyperion theater in Silverlake and it consists of performances of unnerving short fiction, freewheeling choreography, and an editor who has set up a typewriter outside the theater to sell poetry on demand. Ethan buys me a poem and I'm delighted, but also a little worried. This is not the kind of thing he would normally attend unless forced at knifepoint. But as he chats up a different editor, I understand—he's trying to help me want to be alive again.

I exchange contact information with the editor and, later, I submit a short story I wrote from the point-of-view of the second-to-last victim of a serial killer in a horror film. Shortly after it is accepted, the editor sends me an email. He is on the board of an experimental opera company that, in 2013, put together a site-specific, immersive opera at Union Station called *Invisible Cities*. The show received universal critical acclaim and was a finalist for the 2014 Pulitzer Prize. Now they're about to begin developing a new show that will take place at locations across the city. Do I want to meet to discuss joining the team who will write the opera's libretto?

At our meeting, I pitch a story that hinges on multiple iterations of Los Angeles happening on top of one another like branches on a tree. Shortly thereafter I'm signing a contract and sitting in on rehearsals with five other librettists and six composers. A reporter shows up to observe, and a few weeks later, an article about our opera pops up in a local magazine. Features in the *New York Times* and *The New Yorker* follow. Because of the press, the well-known composers, our charismatic director, the shows sell out quickly.

My mother and grandmother fly in from Houston on buddy passes Aunt Tina gets from her job working the customer service phone line at United. I go to pick them up from their hotel to find my mother dressed in a gray T-shirt that is too small for her, her hair uncombed. I try not to mind.

Downtown, we climb into a limousine full of opera singers, one of whom pulls tarot cards and sings our fortunes as we ride. We watch performances that take place under a freeway overpass, in a park, just outside a graveyard, in Little Tokyo and Boyle Heights. Each car's route delves into the opera's central question: whether it is possible to find and name the initial point out of which everything else in this city emerged.

"What's interesting about this to you?" my grandmother leans over to ask me. "Is it just that they sing your words?"

"Sure," I say, as we pull into the Bradbury Building. A woman in a bright red dress steps off the landing, mid-aria, followed by a man in a top hat blowing into a trombone.

"I've always preferred jazz," she whispers back.

My mother, who says that my grandmother has no imagination, is too concrete a thinker to appreciate art, appears truly in awe of the show. She especially loves the music composed by a violinist from Nevada, who makes astonishing, dissonant arrangements, like metal on metal, wild and harsh. I wrote the scenes that feature his compositions.

"People need this kind of beauty in their lives," my mother says. "I'm so proud of you." Our show explores the question of whether or not Los Angeles has a center. I feel then that I have reached the center, that it is here with me and my mother and the performers, exactly where we are.

But she flies home the next day and won't pick up when I call her. Days pass. Then a week. She has gone back to not speaking to me—this much is clear—but what's not clear is why.

"She called me saying you were fawning over one of the girls in the opera," says my grandmother when I call. "The girl who read your tarot cards, I guess. Of course, you can love whoever you want, but she thinks you cheated on Ethan."

There are over 120 singers in the production. I have never actually met the singer my mother seems to think I'm sleeping with. But my mother is usually so good at reading my mind—or she was when I was a child—that I try to rationalize the thought, searching for any circumstance in which she might be telling the truth. Did I cheat on Ethan with this woman and forget about it somehow? How could I have done something so terrible to someone I love?

"Were you not going to mention this to me?" I ask now trying not to let my grandmother hear the anger I feel.

"I didn't want you to be worried," she answers. I can tell the strain in my voice upsets her.

MY MOTHER TEXTS ME SAYING she would not have come to see the show if she knew I was a lesbian. She's angry I'm cheating on Ethan and believes now that I'm a bad person. The leaps of logic in her accusations make it difficult for me to deny what she's saying without feeling as if I'm acting. Ultimately I give up trying, frightened of what her rage does to my sense of reality. I worry I'll give in to her doubt, accidentally slip into an alternate plane.

But the opera is a hit and the director wins a MacArthur "genius grant." A literary agent named Jill reaches out to find out if I have any writing she can sell, and we meet for lunch at a French restaurant on Vermont Avenue in Los Feliz. I tell her I'll be done with *The Anatomy Book* the following year. Months later, when my mother decides she's talking to me again, I simply don't answer the phone. I delete all her email messages without reading them and set up a filter that sends them to spam.

I MISS THE FIRST DEADLINE Jill and I set for *The Anatomy Book*, then the second. I give a partial draft to Ethan, whose incapacity for coddling is total. *Your central character has to make choices!* He writes in the margins. *She can't just think!* And: *We get it, she's depressed, but what is she doing? Where is she in space?* He finishes the notes by telling me bluntly that the book needs to be pulled apart and put back together differently if it's going to get better. He leaves notes for me on the whiteboard on our fridge: revise chapter one, chapter two, chapter three.

"How am I supposed to do this?" I ask.

"Just make a list and cross things off," he says.

"Maybe I should give up," I say.

"Success is what exists on the other side of hard,"[9] Ethan says.

"Did you just make that up?"

"No. It's what Doc Rivers told the Clippers last night."

"And they won?"

"No," he concedes. "But they're all millionaires."

Instead of writing, I return to my affirmations. I have graduated from Dr. Sideroff's CDs to Louise Hay's videos on YouTube. *I am loved. You are loved. I am full of light. You are full of light. I love the world. You love the world.* I listen when I wake up in the morning, when I do laundry, when I get ready for bed, let Louise tell me that I am worth love and that I approve of myself and that I wish for peace for the entire world. Listening, I forgive everyone who has ever hurt me, let all past transgressions float away. I experience moments of intense joy while walking the dog and driving. Then my mother calls. It's been over a year since we last spoke. Buoyed by my affirmations, I decide, for once, to answer.

To my surprise, she tells me she loves me and that she wants to apologize. "I'm sorry," she says. "You were right. About everything. I'm so sorry I hurt you." Half in shock, I listen for an hour before I understand: it's the meditations I've been doing. All my forgiveness. I've filled the world with peace and light and some of it has reached her. What other explanation is there? She asks if she can call me again and I tell her she can. I hang up and tell Ethan what I've accomplished with my affirmations. He says, "Sure, okay, but what about your book? Did you write today?"

He doesn't believe I manifested my mother's call. And if I'm honest, something does seem off. She sounded weird, a little stoned, which is strange because my mother is afraid of drugs and barely even drinks.

I leave a message for my grandmother, just to make sure. She calls me back, and that is when I learn about the cars my mother believes have been following her down the interstate.

THE NIGHT AFTER MY GRANDMOTHER calls, I think back to the writer friend I met at a residency who, after I told her about my mother's reaction to the opera, suggested my mother might have un-diagnosed borderline personality disorder. She sent me an article to read that suddenly made me feel very awake. "Living with a person with BPD is . . . 'like living with Mount Vesuvius always on the verge of erupting,'" the essay's author wrote.[10] And even though she was writing about her mother, it was as if she was writing about mine.

Now, researching whether psychosis is a symptom of BPD, I discover another symptom, apophenia. The term, coined by German psychiatrist Klaus Conrad, refers to a strong feeling that an invisible pattern that governs the world is always just about to reveal itself. I remember then what I felt like in Paris, that sense of overarching certainty that every moment held a clue to some great mystery I was just about to solve. Apophenia, I learn, is a hallmark of schizophrenia.

I read a profile of Jennifer Egan in *The New Yorker* in which Egan speaks about the relationship between schizophrenia and creative production. Her brother, Graham, who suffered from schizophrenia and ultimately committed suicide, sometimes compared the voices he heard in his head to the voices of her characters.

"You're hearing voices and you're making a living from it. And *I'm* hearing voices and spending a fortune trying to get rid of them," he told her.[11] She describes knowing that her life and her brother's life could as easily have been reversed, that her own relative sanity was only a matter of chance. "To be mentally ill is bad luck, and to not be mentally ill is good luck. And in bad moments, I feel so . . . *engulfed* by the violence of his bad luck that I almost feel like I can't function."

There it is again, I think. That word: luck.

FIVE

IN LATE 2017, I FLY home from LAX, land at IAH at midnight, and take a Lyft to my grandmother's condo. The condo looks the same as always: on the walls, paintings of tall, thin African women going to and from market, baskets mounted on their heads. A stalk of raw cotton sits in a vase by the door. The coffee table is draped in patterned mudcloth and covered in books: *Women, Culture & Politics*, by Angela Davis; *The Devil That Danced on the Water*, by Aminatta Forna; a copy of Sadie's debut poetry collection, *Belle Afrique*.

Sadie's profile has skyrocketed and she's become one of the few young poets in the country whose name the general public knows. These days, it is difficult to get her on the phone. She's always traveling or waking up early to be a guest on NPR. At parties, when people learn we are close, they speak about her book in breathless tones: "Oh, I love her." *But you don't even know her*, I always want to say back. *I* love her. She's established a massive following online for her outspokenness and willingness to speak truth to power. My feelings about her newfound fame are complex, and I find myself now covering up my grandmother's copy of her book with a history of the war in Liberia.

Snooping through a cardboard box of files, I discover a manila envelope full of notes from my mother. The notes offer a detailed outline of everything she believes is happening to her, starting with the ever-present white men in sunglasses following her in their big trucks and blocking the door when she tries to go to church. She wrote letters to her pastor, asking for surveillance camera tape so she could take it to the city attorney. In the envelope also are notes my grandmother took detailing the events of the past few months: my mother is walking up and down the street shoeless, in socks, being stopped by the neighbors and looking through them as if she has no idea who they are. I find a letter my grandmother wrote, pleading with my mother to search within herself for signs that things aren't right. On the back of it, my mother has scrawled a response, saying she is going to move out of the neighborhood because she's found a good job. This was the nursing position she would go on to leave one month later because she believed it was part of the intricate plot against her.

I spend all night laying out each item on the floor and taking pictures. Searching for a pattern in her actions that might predict what she will do next. My phone lights up. It's Ethan, sending me a picture of the dog in the bathtub, shampoo making her fur stand on end. She peers at me through the screen, a little pale ghost, and everything about my life there appears impossibly far away.

IN THE MORNING, I LEAVE my grandmother's condo and go to the fourplex in Third Ward where her office used to be and where my mother now stays. She's essentially living in my grandmother's former waiting room and supply room where she has stretched socks along the floorboards and draped a black shirt over the top of the door that leads to the bathroom. A large black desk chair sits in one corner. Otherwise, the room is bare.

I read a book not long ago called *Crazy Like Us*, by Ethan Watters, and learned that people with schizophrenia—the disorder now named and staring up at me starkly from my mother's most recent intake paperwork—tend to fare better in developing countries than in the United States. Some research suggests it's not the treatment here that leads to worse outcomes but the fear of the disease that family members and friends project onto the schizophrenic person.[12] To Americans, schizophrenia is not only frightening, it is an existential threat. "We become abject," writes Juli McGruder, an anthropologist formerly at the University of Puget Sound, "when contemplating mentation that seems more changeable, less restrained and less controllable, more open to outside influence than we imagine our own to be."[13]

Having read this, I want to say I approach my mother with love and understanding—I want to be the type of person who approaches a situation like this with love and understanding—but McGruder is correct. I only feel despair.

"It's so empty," I say lightly.

"I had a roach infestation," my mother says. She looks so thin, and her eyes are so bright she reminds me of a little girl. I want to take her somewhere and feed her and keep her warm. "Bugs all in my things."

She tells me she is sorry she couldn't come get me from the airport. She had to stay in the room to protect her chair. She sleeps in it.

"I don't want to have to sleep on the floor," she tells me. "It's so cold."

I ask her whom she needs to protect her chair from.

"My life," she says, "has become very strange lately."

She tells me she applied for a job at a local college, but to get it she has to send in all her old college transcripts, and she can't seem to lay her hands on them.

"What kind of job?" I ask.

"Dean of Student Services," she says. "I like working with students and helping them."

"I think you need a certain amount of experience for that kind of job. Possibly a PhD."

She considers this, then her face breaks open into a smile and she tells me about the day she and my dad got married. "It was a really beautiful day," she says, "March twenty-first, nineteen eighty-five." It's the first time she's ever told me anything about her marriage to my dad without my asking, and the way she describes it, I can see her, barely out of her teens and not knowing anything yet about the future, four months pregnant with me.

"I wore a dress I got from one of our trips to Mexico. Just a white dress I wore every day. After we got married, we went to your dad's mother's house and she cooked for everybody. I was really happy, at least right then. It was a really good day." Her voice turns sardonic, though her smile stays put. "That was one thing your dad is good for. He sure could marry somebody."

I no longer remember what it was like to live with my dad, only his early visits to Houston from Oakland. I'd perch on his shoulders clutching the stuffed animal he'd brought me while we walked to the park. He stopped coming when my mother sued him for child support. As a child when I got in trouble and was being punished, I cried out for him, until I overheard my mother tell my grandmother it worried her, as my dad was gone and not coming back. After that, I started screaming that I wanted my mother when I was being scolded, even when she was the one doing the scolding, because when it came to choosing sides, it felt crucial to choose hers, even at the expense of myself.

She remedied the problem ingeniously by teaching me to cry with my mouth closed. I was allowed to throw tantrums when I needed to, but I was not allowed to make any noise.

"I can check my email!" my mother says now from the other side of the room, sounding delighted. She clutches her phone in her hand. "I haven't been able to check my email in months!"

"What do you mean?" I ask, wary, trying not to show it.

"It was like someone reached down through the internet and took away all my email! It was being held hostage. Now my password is working. Maybe you're my good-luck charm!"

She turns to the window and tells me about the too-loud cars that go whooshing by every night. "You would not believe the noise," she says, pained. She picks up a bent black plastic straw from a child's juice box and shows it to me, tells me it is her toothbrush. When I ask her, again, what she means, she sighs.

"Long story."

Ethan texts me. How is everything? The text is followed by a series of pictures of the dog in the bathtub again.

Cute. How are you guys?

Why didn't you answer my question?

Everything is fine.

You're lying. I can tell.

I put my phone away.

My mother is telling me again about Lance Blanks, how he is stalking her and how she wrote a letter of complaint to something she calls the "Internet Board." She is cracking up while she speaks, laughing the way you laugh in a nightmare or when you're coming out of a dream where everything was funny but you can't remember why.

"Oh Lord, I don't know. All I can do is listen to his voice and try my best to stay sane. He won't let me sleep . . . Lance . . . he won't let me sleep."

"Does Lance sometimes tell you to break things?" I ask.

"I smashed up some cars and broke some glass," she admits. But then she says they were only dummy cars, put there to bait her. The police came, and the next thing she knew she was being tased and she was in the hospital again. No one told me she'd been tased, and I wonder if she only thinks she was or if this fact was hidden from me.

"Lance had me believing Granny was trying to kill me. That she had sold me into sex slavery. I couldn't understand it. I was scared. I kept trying to explain it to her, and she would look at me like I was crazy." She is getting upset, so I change the subject.

"Getting rid of all your stuff was probably a good move," I say. "Now you can have a fresh start."

"Yes," she says after a pause, as if she's suddenly realizing I am slow. "It is a good idea to get rid of all your stuff when it's infested with roaches."

"How do you feel now?" I ask.

"Feel?" she says, almost shrieking. "How am I supposed to feel?"

By now it's late afternoon and the light is fading, darkness taking up all the space in the room. It feels urgent that I run away before we are both submerged. Feeling my face wobble, I stand up and ready myself to go. She watches me as I leave and under the weight of her stark glare I feel like a criminal.

BEFORE I LEFT, MY MOTHER gave me a notebook. In it she's listed the makes and models of all the white cars following her, along with the direction they were headed in and/or where they were parked. Her entries are analytical, thorough and precise, repetitive and dense. All of the entries are dated. The days don't proceed chronologically but move back and forth between January 13 and March 13. She writes that one hundred people follow her in cars twenty-four hours a day with their headlights on, honking, and that police officers refuse to help. She also keeps her own detailed medical notes:

Mon, March 13, 11–12 pm, Lance lasered the left cranium (back) repeatedly. I told him how badly it hurt several times. He responded by continuing to laser me in the same spot all night. I walked, jumped, squatted, throughout the evening and night to avoid the laser. He has told me that he pushed a powder through and placed it on my teeth. So my teeth are permanently blue now. He has explained to me that I will need dental work and the placement of thin veneers.

Under this report, she has scribbled the address of a local dentist, his name, and directions to his office. Then a new note:

I am on my sixth day of not eating solid food. [Lance] is pushing air in my stomach, alternatingly with layering my left back skull. He said he could see me naked and he constantly made terribly lewd remarks. He said he watches my mother and sister naked. He says he has inserted cameras into my eyes and around the house.

In the notebook, she details a litany of abuse: microphones and speakers placed in her teeth, sensors all over her body, her DNA analyzed, the roof of her mouth sloughed off, sterility due to a diaphragm Lance placed inside her secretly, loud airplane noises overhead, all parts of his scheme to force her to appear on a reality show, which began years before.

She writes out the rules of the show:

A day of starvation consists of not having eaten a morsel of food. There can be no more than three days of starvation. There can only be one eight-day period of starvation per year. A morsel is a complex protein—for example, one bean.

I read the notebook to my grandmother as we eat lunch outside at a Mediterranean restaurant on West Alabama. The air around us is gritty with the sand crossing over the Atlantic from the Sahara that the wind brings to Houston every few seasons. I tell her what I'm thinking: if only we can figure out where the problem started, then maybe we can arrive at a solution.

But my grandmother insists my mother can fix herself. That she's choosing not to. "She has to reach inside herself and find some kind of strength," she says. "She'll do it when she hits rock bottom."

How is this not rock bottom? I wonder. Shifting into safer territory, I ask her who is going to pay the bill for the nights my mother has been spending in the emergency room, which I imagine are expensive. She lets out a sigh.

"Black people don't worry about debt," she says. "Black people worry about getting food to eat, getting a place to stay. That's what Black people worry about." She shakes her head. "The way we live is below working-class."

"You don't live below working-class," I say. If she were anybody else, I would be confused by the sudden change in topic, but my grandmother always finds her way back to the Struggle.

"I say 'we,' but I pay all my bills on time," she concedes. "I'm sure if your mother got bunches of money she would pay her bills."

"How would she get bunches of money?" I ask.

"That's how white people pay their bills!" she says. "They get bunches of money. Black people are having a hard time. We have been made a permanent underclass in this country—"

I repeat to my grandmother, whom I suspect now is trying to change the subject, what my mother told me, that she thinks she's in a competition to be married off to Lance Blanks. She thinks my grandmother knows this but isn't acknowledging it. This lack of acknowledgment scares her and makes her angry because she believes my grandmother is in on the plot against her.

"One thing you could do if you wanted," I say, "is you could say, 'Oh, I'm sorry that's happening to you, oh, that's terrible.' You could gain her trust by listening instead of reacting to what she is telling you."

"I don't know," she says.

"What don't you know?"

"It seems like it would hurt to be in on the delusions."

"But you're not supporting the delusion, you're supporting the way she feels. Instead of saying, 'You're not sick, you need to get it together,' you say, 'Oh, it must be so frightening to think that, you must be so scared.'"

"I haven't had the chance to talk to your mother about Lance," she says, as if the problem is one of scheduling and not psychosis.

"But you don't have to talk to her about it. Just acknowledge something is wrong."

"I don't understand what's going on in her brain. She took a hammer and broke out the windows on the neighbors' cars."

"I know. I told you, Lance told her those cars weren't real."

"All those police cars showed up and—"

"It doesn't even matter what you say! Memorize a line. Repeat it. You don't even have to mean it."

"I think well or ill, your mother does not like me."

"It's not about you—"

"But I'm a part of whatever this is. She doesn't trust me."

"She doesn't distrust you. She thinks it's Lance making you ignore her, so if you could—"

"When you were growing up, I was always the object of distrust."

"That's true. But not like this."

I pause, sit back in my chair, collect myself, try to reset. "This must be exhausting for you," I say. "It must be so hard. Are you getting any help?"

"You know, sometimes I think, If I ever let myself start to cry," she says, "I would never stop."

"But that's depression," I say. "That's what therapy is for."

She rolls her eyes. "Black people don't go to therapy," she says. "Black people fake it 'til they make it."

On the drive home we pass a hunched unhoused woman with a ragged scarf knotted around her head. My grandmother points.

"She must have decided to go for a walk."

That can't be her, I think. But when we catch up to her and I see the woman's face, I am startled to discover she is right.

It's true my grandmother is a poster child for faking it until you make it. She had a debilitatingly depressed mother and a violent, abusive husband. Now she's a successful small business owner who travels the world. Of course she's in denial. Denial is how she survived. I also faked it, more or less, or am faking it, and someday I too hope to make it. Still, I do not believe my mother is going to be able to fake it until she makes it out of this.

SIX

IN *THE ARCADES PROJECT*, BENJAMIN quotes the French revolutionary Louis Auguste Blanqui, who wrote that everything happening to us now is also happening on planets identical to ours that we will never see. In infinite versions of this world, the same events play out eternally with no change or improvement. "The universe repeats itself endlessly and paws the ground in place."[14] Before Benjamin died, inspired by a painting by his friend Paul Klee, he would describe history as an angel whose "face is turned toward the past."

"Where a chain of events appears to us," this angel "sees one single catastrophe which keeps piling wreckage upon wreckage and hurls it in front of his feet."[15]

I read an article in the *Atlantic* suggesting children born to Black single mothers are the least likely of all children to achieve upward mobility, and a different article, in the *Washington Post*, comparing the average net worth of Black families in America ($17,600) to that of white families ($171,000).[16] I wonder a little bitterly whether it occurs to the people who write these articles, some of whom are Black themselves, that the daughters of Black single mothers will read them, or that we read at all, or if we pass in front of everyone else at a wavelength no one else perceives.

Because if the researchers are right and if inheritance determines our destinies, and if Benjamin is right and our fates are fixed and terrible, then how does anyone do anything? Are we all lying to ourselves all the time? I remind myself Benjamin was writing in exile, persecuted and soon to be stateless, at the dawn of World War II. His brother died in a concentration camp. He nearly died in one, too. Underlying much of his late writing was the conviction that a world in which progress was automatic, in which things simply got better as time passed, was not a world that would ever produce the Europe in which he lived.

But I need to believe progress is possible—if not, what is the point of writing my book? Or trying to help my mother? Benjamin might reply that there is no point, that freedom from history is the only goal, and it is one we will never accomplish. Or, as he writes quoting Kafka in conversation with his friend Max Brod: "Oh, plenty of hope, an infinite amount of hope—but not for us."[17]

AUNT TINA COMES OVER TO my grandmother's condo and together the three of us watch an episode of a cooking competition show called *Chopped*. When the only Black contestant wins with his stew of okra, tomatoes, and onions, we cheer. My grandmother frowns.

"What's wrong?" Aunt Tina says. "He won!"

"Ten thousand dollars!" I say. "He'll finally be able to open his food truck."

"He wouldn't have to cook food on TV if white people hadn't brought us over on boats in the first place," my grandmother says.

"He would be back home in Africa with the rest of his people, happy and free."

"Can't argue with that," Aunt Tina says, grabbing her purse and nodding at me that it's time to go. She wants to check out a new wine bar she thinks I'll like in the upscale neighborhood where I went to school. Granny declines to join. At an outdoor table, over cocktail samosas and a flight of pink wines, Tina asks if Ethan and I are ever going to get married.

"What if I'm afraid to get married?" I say, and what I mean is, What about when what happened to my mother happens again? To me? Or what if it skips me but lands on whatever child I may or may not have?

Aunt Tina levels a pointed gaze at me. "Schizophrenia is not a death sentence. Your mom would get better if she would go to a doctor and take meds. But she won't."

"I wonder if maybe Granny could convince her to do that."

Aunt Tina rolls her eyes. "You know how Granny is." What she means is, my grandmother, having watched her mother die of breast cancer, distrusts doctors implicitly, believes hospitals are only in it for the money, has in common with my mother the belief that the second any one of us succumbs to taking a prescription drug, we've signed our own death warrant.

I wonder if Aunt Tina or my grandmother ever says, "You know how Sarah is," and if they do, what it is they mean when they say that.

"Anyway," she says, "don't be scared. Marriage means being there. It's a promise one person makes to be around."

It's true Ethan and I have never had the kind of love that has us constantly saying nice things to each other. We have the kind that keeps us consistently in each other's lives. If one of us calls, the other always picks up or calls back seconds later; if one of us is stuck in a boring conversation, the other can always be relied upon to come to the rescue. If one of us feels like lying down in the road, the other listens and explains why nothing is ever that bad. And this, I think, and have always thought, is somehow better than what other couples have.

But it's true also that I've followed in my mother's footsteps in other ways. We are both quiet and slow to trust others, insular and insecure. The psychologist Resmaa Menakem writes about the embodiment of experience passed down to us, how some memories are handed down not in the form of words but through our skin and our nervous system in ways that bypass language. Menakem writes, "You can think one thing, and your body can simultaneously respond as if you had exactly the opposite thought."[18] Not everything we do or say has conscious origins, and much of what drives our behavior is invisible.

"Tell me about Lance Blanks," I say to Aunt Tina. I've been looking him up on my phone periodically. He appears to be a nice, well-to-do former professional athlete, the father of two girls he loves very much.

She remembers he was in tenth grade when my mother was a senior at James Madison High School. He was a varsity basketball player, and they used to go to his games, their whole group of friends piling into my mother's car. "He had a crush on your mom. He was funny. He liked to play around. I don't think I ever once saw him sad." She smiles. "He was goofy like me."

"And what was my mom like then? Was there any sign of what's happening to her now?"

"Remember how when you were a little kid, when she punished you, she used to put you in the closet? You know, I didn't know about then, but I guess your mother must have mentioned it to Granny at some point—"

"It wasn't that bad when she put me in the closet," I say. "The apartment was small. I was loud. Where else was I supposed to go?"

"You better either shut it up or go in the closet," my aunt says, doing an imitation of my angry mother, and I laugh. "Anyway, I remember the day after Granny told us our daddy died, she had to go away for a business trip. She said we didn't have to go to school if we didn't want to. Left us at home with the babysitter. Your mama went into her closet and stayed there for twenty-four hours."

In her book *Understanding the Borderline Mother*, Christine Ann Lawson writes, "Unbearable pain that is expressed and acknowledged becomes bearable. But borderlines received no such responses in their childhood. Therefore, they are stuck in the past, trying to elicit what they needed as a child—validation of their unbearable pain."[19]

My mother is fourteen. She learns her father is dead. Her mother leaves. She goes to sit alone in her closet. No one comes to explain what happened or why it happened or to tell her she'll be okay.

"She always had a temper," my aunt says now. "She stopped speaking to me for a whole year after you graduated college. She never told me why. Then one day she called and left me a voice-mail saying she wasn't mad anymore. That I could come see her if I wanted." She tells me about other incidents: my mother crashing her car on purpose into the garage door of a man she was dating whom she suspected of cheating. Calls to my grandmother from other ex-boyfriends, asking her to please call my mother off. I imagine my mother doing those things and then imagine her still in her closet, stuck there, even now, waiting for help that won't ever come.

"What about your dad?" I ask. "Did Granny ever mention anything about mental illness?"

"He had this same anger thing. Threw acid on a little white girl at his school when she tried to touch his science experiment. Ended up having to graduate in juvenile detention. You know that story?"

I do. On the rare occasions when my grandmother talks about my grandfather, it's only ever to tell me the same two facts: he got kicked out of high school for throwing acid on a white girl who touched his science experiment, and when he started at the University of Texas, he faked a British accent and told everyone he was a Nigerian prince.

But, Tina says, she doesn't remember anybody ever saying he had anything like paranoia or schizophrenia. "We didn't think in terms of people having mental illnesses. That didn't happen to people you knew."

When her own father died, my mother went into the closet and stayed there for a day. When I was little and did something to make her angry, she put me in the closet and told me I could not come out. She might have been reenacting her own trauma, giving me a loss to match hers. Attempting to take control of life's ruthlessness by creating a reality for me that felt familiar to her. Sustaining her grief in me. Who's to say I won't do the same? To my own future child or to anyone who loves me? Who's to say people aren't patterns that repeat forever in everything like the branching shapes of trees?

"Why am I doing this?" I ask Ethan when I'm home again, back to staring in misery at my manuscript. "Why even write?"

"To make life better for other people," he responds.

I look at him and wonder what it feels like to move through the world as if destiny is not a force to be wrestled into submission but rather a relative whose love one both takes for granted and returns. What is it like to be fine?

SADIE CALLS WHILE I'M WALKING to the laundromat carrying a bag of my clothes. She tells me she'll be passing through L.A. soon to give a poetry lecture at USC. I tell her about my visit to see my mother, and when she asks me how I feel, I say okay, actually. I don't know. I can't feel anything. I have, in the week since I returned, grown numb.

"You know not being able to engage emotionally could be damaging in the long run, right?" Sadie prods. "Or do you think it helps you in some way, not feeling things?"

Memories like movie stills: in middle school, when my best friend Allison told me, sobbing, in front of the gym, that her parents were getting divorced, I stopped speaking to her entirely, let her second-best friend replace me, and gradually shifted into a different friend group altogether.

When I worked at the French bakery in high school, I saw a little girl break a glass, cut herself, and start to bleed. I stared into space, frozen, until her grandmother practically swung at me. "Can you help us? A little girl is hurt," she shouted. Afterward my coworkers looked at me strangely and I had no explanation for my behavior. When bad things happened in front of me, I went somewhere else.

Annoyed, I change the subject to *The Anatomy Book*. Sadie asks

me if I think I'll finish it soon. I say I have to. That everything depends on it. "Either that or I'll try to become an influencer," I say.
"Don't those people make money hand over fist?"

The silence that follows is tinged with alarm, as if I've said
something deeply offensive.

"I'm kidding," I say.

"Good. We're not *young* anymore," she says, and I know enough
not to get my feelings hurt. Sadie believes in absolute transparency.
There's something attractive about her utter inability to bullshit.
Her total lack of fear in the face of confrontation. And anyway, as
always, she's right.

In the novel I'm struggling to write, a version of Sadie appears
as Parker, the protagonist's roommate. She is the wealthy daughter of an Eritrean doctor father and a white mother and, also like
Sadie, was educated mostly abroad, and so speaks with an accent
that weighs down every word she says with gravitas. Parker wants
fundamentally to be respected, while Laura wants fundamentally
to be liked. Parker's approach to life has gotten her further. Laura's
approach, up to the point at which the events of the book take
place, has kept her safe.

I FEED MY LAUNDRY INTO the washing machine and go for a walk
while it runs. Los Feliz is bordered by a growing tent city, and the
people who live there are familiar to me, though I don't know
their names. I pass the tall white man who wears oversized shorts
and a gray hoodie and a skullcap even in the months when the
sky blazes so hot, it is as if a layer of the ozone is missing; the two

Black women, one young, one old, who sit on a blanket and shout cheerfully at everyone who passes; the blue-eyed white woman who could be the mother of one of my friends except that she never speaks or makes eye contact and always has with her a shopping cart full of her things.

The people who live in and around the tent city in my neighborhood show up in *The Anatomy Book* as the SEO, or the Society for the Eternality of Objects. Those in the SEO believe that, in the same way newspapers, hardcover books, videotapes, and photographs have become relics of a dark age, humans, too, might be lost to the passage of time. They sleep on the New York City streets and eschew technology in favor of tangible objects, trying to save the physical world from erasure by holding on to the things we can touch.

In the book, others urge them to grasp that their world already has ended, that they have no choice but to step out into the weightless new one where everyone lives now, but the people in the SEO disagree. They stage terrorist attacks as a form of resistance, blowing up various buildings while the more artistic among them engage in street theater to distract the police.

I pass Jennifer, the elderly woman who sleeps outside the neighborhood bookstore and has lived in the area much longer than I have. Whenever I see her she is singing or shouting or dancing with her blanket. If she is not doing one of these things, she is asleep. A trait common to the less lucid unhoused people who live in my neighborhood is that, like my mother, they display chaotic levels of emotion. And it's true—Sadie is right—that a long time ago I adopted my grandmother's practice of total removal as the healthiest way to approach the world and not be poisoned by it. My dispassion, like hers, is also an act of self-preservation.

MY GRANDMOTHER CALLS TO TELL me a neighbor had to call the police on my mother the night before. She was standing outside in a bathing suit, no shoes, screaming at passersby. This neighbor has known her for twenty years. But now when she tries to approach her, my mother curses and threatens her.

JAMES BALDWIN'S STEPFATHER FLEW INTO rages. Punished his children for no reason. Alienated his sisters. Suffered from a deep paranoia. Locked himself up alone and moaned and sang, believing he could communicate with the Lord. But because he was a preacher, it was only when he stopped eating, having accused Baldwin's mother of trying to poison him, that the family understood something was wrong. He was committed and died, of tuberculosis, in the hospital, still refusing food.

Even after the root of his dad's illness was uncovered, Baldwin was afraid he would inherit it and that it would kill him. He attributed this fear to an "intolerable bitterness of spirit,"[20] which he himself developed during a summer working in a defense plant in New Jersey in 1942. He was banned from an all-white lunch counter, laughed at, followed, and fired from his job three times. The repetition of the phrase "We don't serve Negroes here" drove him to feel his life was in danger from the hatred he carried in his own heart.

"Between pity and guilt and fear I began to feel that there was another me trapped in my skull like a jack-in-the-box who might escape my control at any moment and fill the air with screaming," he wrote. He lived in fear of this other self because he knew hatred, which could destroy so much, "never failed to destroy the man who hated." He likens his sense of having to contain it to a blind fever that would never be cured.

ETHAN WANTS TO KNOW WHY my grandmother can't put my mother in an institution. What are we supposed to do, I say, re-home her like a stray cat? Where would we even put her? There are no public mental institutions, haven't been since Reagan pulled their funding and they all shut down in the '80s. Also, she has rights. If she doesn't want to get help, no one can make her. The most any psychiatric ward will do is hold her for a few days until she is deemed, by some arbitrary, inaccurate metric, to no longer be a danger to herself and other people.

Ethan's father sends me a list of psychiatrists in Houston who might be able to help. One by one, they offer their apologies but say they can't talk to me about my mother due to HIPAA laws. But one recommends NAMI, the National Alliance on Mental Illness, and its network of support groups.

The NAMI group I join meets in the recreation room of a nursing home in Sherman Oaks, California. Some of the residents have pets, and I watch little dogs keep pace behind their masters across the lobby carpet. An old man with a walker wanders into our classroom twice. Each time, he turns around after a minute or two and pushes himself back out, unimpressed.

Across the world, we learn—from China to Colombia to the Czech Republic to Denmark to India to Russia to the UK—people with schizophrenia present the same symptoms: lack of insight into their condition, paranoia, unwillingness to cooperate, false ideas, emotional dullness, poor rapport, and auditory hallucinations. In the U.S., African Americans are four times more likely to be diagnosed with schizophrenia than Caucasians. Latinos are more than three times more likely, though both statistics may be the result of a tendency to overdiagnose the disorder in minority populations.

The group is run by three volunteers: a youngish, pink-faced man, immaculately dressed with a wave of blond hair, who tells us he has a brother who is homeless by choice; a nurse married to a woman who routinely destroys their apartment in fits of rage that she does not later remember; and an old man in a baseball cap who doesn't explain his relationship to the program but only gazes at us tiredly.

I learn certain events can trigger illnesses in anyone's brain that would have otherwise lain dormant for the patient's entire lifetime. At any point, any one of us might take a wrong turn and tip over into a false reality. A wrong marriage, a bad breakup, a mix-up at the DMV, and our lives might be different forever. The lives of our children as well. Most unfair of all is the condition called anosognosia, which makes it impossible for the person suffering to recognize they have a disease. It leads to a fundamental lack of trust in those who want to help, since any suggestion of mental illness is perceived as an attack. Later, the tired-looking man tells us his wife lost her sanity after a disastrous camping trip.

Someone hands out pictures of brain scans on which chunks of gray matter have been circled and labeled with arrows. I search them

NO ONE GETS TO FALL APART

for a lesion where schizophrenia is, a wound an expert might shine a light on and heal, but the arrows appear to be pointing at nothing.

BEFORE THE GROUP STARTED, WE each signed up via email for a night to bring dinner. That first night, a woman from Glendale whose brother thinks the CEO of Disney is talking to him through the radio unveils a container of pulled pork, a vat of three-layer dip from Gelson's, baklava, and spinach puffs. The room fills with the smell of cheese and dough. People gather around the trays and help themselves to glasses of lemonade. The point of the meal is for us to mingle. But I can't help noticing I'm the only Black person here. We'd each received a binder full of information about mental illness diagnoses, and though whoever wrote it was careful to account for differences across cultures, it's still clear that whiteness is the default from which every other diagnosis deviates. I consider not coming back, not certain how any of the questions I have can be answered in this room.

But after dinner, the others share more intimate stories about their loved ones: The son with major clinical depression who will no longer play music at his nephew's birthday parties. The brother who lives in a tent in Elysian Park and chain-smokes because it eases the symptoms. The daughter who has twice been arrested for walking barefoot and naked up the middle of the street. The child who is in and out of UCLA's psychiatric hospital since the onset of a psychotic episode triggered by cannabis. The sister who got in bed one day and won't get out. As we finish going around the room, we end with the story of a woman's daughter who is looking into assisted suicide. The mother, who is sitting next to me, says she doesn't blame her, then cuts herself off as she starts to cry. By the end of class, I've learned that if one of my parents has schizophrenia, I have a 13 percent chance of getting it. But the binder doesn't tell me what my chances are of giving it to my child, should I have one. I decide I will keep coming back to the support group, if only to find out whether the people in the class who have sick children are glad they have them anyway, and if, given the choice, they would have them again.

We share what we do for a living. I tell the group about a freelance writing project I've been working on for the past year, a libretto for a choral piece commissioned by the California Chorus, the house choir at Walt Disney Concert Hall in downtown L.A. The piece is called *Manifest Destinies*, and it takes on the frontier myth in the South from the Reconstruction era to the oil boom to the modern space age. The point, I say, is to make it clear that every boom leads to a bust because we take human nature with us wherever we go. When I realize everyone in the room is staring at me blankly, I stop talking then say, "I also work in fundraising." I describe the day job I recently quit in the university advancement office, and we move on. I feel deeply embarrassed, but relieved, at least, that I did not also bring up my novel.

THE NEXT MORNING, I HAVE coffee with my screenwriter friend Henry, who wants to talk about *The Anatomy Book*. He likes the idea behind it and wants, almost more than I do, for me to pull it off successfully. He's offered to read the latest draft. He has some notes.

"There's a lot of Continental philosophy in here," Henry says. He doesn't say it like it is a good thing.

"It's so hard," I say. "How could anything be this hard?"

"You don't get to quit because it's hard."

But, Henry says, why is the main character always so sad? And maybe the book could do with a little more action? And, even if writing works out, what will I do for money? Henry gets paid a lot to write screenplays, and, though he wants to be a novelist, it shocks him how little authors make. Have I ever considered writing a television pilot?

"No," I tell him. "I'm not writing to get rich. I'm writing to make life better for other people."

"No, you're not," Henry says, which is true. "What do you mean for this book to be about? Who is it for?"

The Anatomy Book is about time travel, I consider saying back. As you know. As for who it's for, that's a question worth considering. But not now. Right now I have to write. After Henry leaves the café, I activate my internet blocker and turn my computer, phone, and iPad off so I won't see any texts. I try almost immediately, automatically, to check my email, and am gratified when I realize I can't.

I open my manuscript and write a chapter in which the graduate student, Mark, explains to Laura how Nicholas Canton, in attempting to go back in time and prevent his execution, discovers there is no escape from his own death. No matter how he tries to change the past, he is always captured, imprisoned, and killed, delivered each time in a different manner to an identical fate. I send the latest draft of the novel to my agent, Jill, in New York. Let's get on the phone, she writes back. I can tell from the tone of the email she's unhappy.

On the phone, she tells me she doesn't believe in Mark and Laura's relationship. The entire plot is predicated on Laura's feelings for Mark, but Mark is something of a black hole, and in reality, he seems like a creep. It's unclear why Laura even wants to help him find Canton's missing work. "Why is she doing this? What does she actually want?"

"I think she believes if she finds Canton's book then it will save her from all the other bad things in her life. But then it turns out, like, the book itself is another bad thing."

Jill is silent, and in her silence I sense her nervousness and her hope. My inability to write a novel that lives up to the potential she saw in me is turning out to be difficult for us both. I'm not ready to admit it, but I'm starting to understand the mistake I made with this draft. There is a piece missing. An emotional core for the writing and the plot to wrap themselves around. I've become so fixated on not allowing myself to go crazy, I've lost touch with the feelings that the story needs to work. This hollow core is epitomized in Mark.

"What if you wrote about your mother?" Jill suggests. But I can't. I don't know how. Like other people who spent too much time reading as children, I grew up thinking of myself as a person in a story, all plot twists and climaxes and reversals of fortune that remained under the purview of some distant narrative force into whose hands my life had been placed. I can't find a logical thread in it for what is happening to my mother. Her illness is unfolding according to no rules at all, and no matter how I try to hold it together, the structure falls to pieces.

SEVEN

IN EARLY 2016, THE COMPOSER Reese Blake hired me to write the libretto for a forty-minute oratorio. I met Reese when we worked together on *Hopscotch*, the experimental immersive opera I co-wrote in 2015. We spent last year and into 2017 working with a researcher from Yale, Morgan Nash, developing our piece about the evolution of the American dream across time and the Western frontier.

Reese grew up in Oak Ridge, Tennessee, and her extended family is from Memphis. One afternoon she calls to tell me in the course of our research she's learned her favorite great-aunt worked for a company named for E. H. Crump, the Memphis mayor from 1910–1915 who helped eradicate Memphis's thriving Black upper-middle class. The rise of this community during the Reconstruction Era and its subsequent destruction under Jim Crow make up our oratorio's first movement. Reese is surprised by how little awareness she had about her own ancestors' relationship to this period of history and wonders what else she doesn't know. We decide we'll record an interview, for use in the libretto, in which she talks openly about the things she might be blind to in her own family's past.

I hang up feeling sad. My work on this project, though I'm proud of it, feels, somehow, dishonest. I'm being paid to make art about how everything we forget repeats itself, and how what we remember makes us who we are. But I am starting at such odds with and at such a remove from my own history and my own family that sometimes making progress on the libretto—imbuing it with emotion and making it into an honest, authentic experience for the listener—feels like building a balance beam over an abyss. I'm blind to something vital in myself and, as with my novel, that blindness is making the writing feel empty.

Fourteen years before, in 2003, St. John's held an end-of-year tea party to which all students and parents in the senior class were invited. The morning of the party, I wore a floral dress from J. Crew, and my mother wore too-tight pants and a shiny top from a discount store called Clothestime. When my grandmother came to pick us up in her Mercedes to drive us to the party, I began to cry.

"What?" My mother scowled, looking at me. Her spandex blouse shone in the sun in ways that looked all wrong.

"I can't go." I waited for her to be mad.

"Come on, Sarah," my grandmother said. I wouldn't move. Finally, she said I could do what I wanted and left. My mother took me to the International House of Pancakes, her favorite place to eat. "Of course you didn't want to go up to that school with all them white people," she said. "I don't know what Granny was thinking."

She read the moment as a triumph. As if I'd chosen her. But the truth was I couldn't trust her not to humiliate me. I was embarrassed to be around her and worried she would undo all the work I'd put in at school over the last twelve years. At the restaurant, as I watched her dip a forkful of hash browns in ketchup, I felt a sense of disgust. Hash browns were not a food for an adult. I needed to keep her separate from my real life if I was ever going to get away.

And last year, in 2016, when Reese, Morgan, and I went to Houston for a week to gather research material for our piece, I did not tell my mother I was coming home. She still doesn't know I was there. Instead, on the day we arrived, I drove the others in the rain to Texas City to visit the BP refinery, which looked like the surface of an alien planet. Cranes pumped and towers puffed and burned and sent out a smell that followed us down the highway. We rode to Galveston, to the beach, where the decommissioned barge we'd planned to visit was closed, leaving us to stand at the water's edge and peer out at the active oil rigs still and ominous on the horizon.

I showed them Houston as I knew it: streets lined with mansions owned by celebrity megachurch pastors and Saudi billionaires, a James Turrell sculpture on Rice University's campus built to align perfectly with the view of the sunset, the old house on Parkwood in Riverside Terrace with its flagstones and big backyard. I spent the week feeling outside of myself, trying to be vigilant, as I assiduously avoided anywhere my mother might be. I did not talk about her, and when they asked to meet my family, I made excuse after excuse.

One night, working late transcribing an interview at a café, I felt the pressure of someone's gaze on the back of my neck. My breath quickened. *My mother*, I remember thinking. *She knows I'm here.* But when I looked up, I saw not my mother but a thirtysome-thing man downloading an image of a Confederate flag and mak-ing it his desktop background, angling his laptop toward me, as if to make sure I could see it. He was wearing New Balance sneakers, a brand that had recently been declared by the Neo-Nazi website *The Daily Stormer* the official shoes of white people, because the company had praised Donald Trump's trade policy.

Watching him, I felt almost as if this man was following a script, acting out the part of "white-supremacist" as assigned to him by social media. Part of me wanted to laugh, to tell him when it came to drive-by psychological abuse, he could not hold a candle to my mother. If anything, as I frantically scribbled down a description of the scene, I felt glad for the material.

Anyway, what I know now about the timeline of schizophrenia leads me to suspect that during that visit, my mother may have been in the prodromal phase, the long stretch of time after psy-chosis becomes imminent but before it has made itself visible. If I'd visited her then on that trip home—a point when, Tina told me later, she'd stopped speaking to Tina and my grandmother and spent all her time alone—and tried to convince her to get help before it was too late, if I'd helped her face her own history, we could perhaps have escaped the past together. Instead, I left her there the way I'm always leaving, the way I am not sure, even now, I want to stop.

UNIVERSITY OF CALIFORNIA–IRVINE OFFERS TO host a workshop performance of our oratorio, a way for us to hear the piece in full before the premiere at Walt Disney Concert Hall. The university choir will sing it and we'll watch their performance and fix what needs fixing before the actual debut.

In a campus rehearsal room, the choir director raises his arms. The room explodes into sound. The music works its way through the air like a purifying force. Writing with Reese means constant exposure to the layer of beauty that lies under everything we can see.

The choir sings lines I collaged from the interviews we did in Houston:

We explored the depths of the Earth.
We found glorious fields.
Oil was where we made our money.
Fancy cars, swimming pools, water-skis, fine dining, fishing
boat, picket fence, deer lease.
Oil was where we made our money.

At the feet of a soprano seated in the front is a sleeping baby. In time to the music, she rocks the baby's carrier back and forth with her foot. Watching, I can't help but think of my mother, young, also in college, and only months away from having me.

My mother once told me that when my grandmother found out she was pregnant, she told her not to come back home with a baby. My mother tried to get an abortion but wound up jumping barefoot off the operating table at the last minute and running out into the street. My dad took her to his parents' house and they decided to get married.

"Barefoot?" a friend asked when I told her that story. "Is that really what happened? Or is that what she told you?" A reminder that I was forever forgetting there might be a difference.

ON A TEN-YEAR-OLD MACBOOK, I have a transcript of an interview I did with my mother for a memoir writing class I took in college. Back at my apartment in Los Feliz, I plug it in, and it whirrs to life with audible distress. In the interview, I'm asking her about her father.

"Why do you need to know?" she asks.

"I'm writing about you."

"What are you going to write?"

"I'm not sure yet."

"Something bad?"

"No, Mom."

"You know, Sarah, I know things weren't perfect. But I did the best I could. I had certain philosophies about parenting that didn't involve me being your friend."

"I know. Tell me about your father."

She says he wore big gold nugget rings and walked around like a gangster, like he knew he was the shit. She remembers a basketball game he took her to: all of a sudden, everybody in the bleachers hit the ground because somebody had a gun. Another time, he picked up her and her sister and told them he was kidnapping them.

"You think of it as romantic," she says, "but later you realize he was trying to rile up your mother. He only drove us around the corner."

She remembers his motorcycle, a Thunderbird. One year they rode it to a carnival in a public park and he entered her in a beauty contest. She won forty dollars and a little green suitcase. "He took the money, but he let me keep the suitcase. And I was so happy. I was just so happy. It was so pretty to look at. It had a little mirror in the top."

Then when he died, she says, "it was all blown back in my face. I still don't know if he killed himself or somebody killed him. But I've thought about it over and over, wondering why, if we had good memories together, he would put himself in a position to be killed. If he ever loved me or if it was all just kind of a fantasy."

She says, "Sarah, your granny told us our father died, and she never mentioned it again. And I never asked her about it. I didn't feel like my mother cared about me. But that wasn't her fault. She didn't know how to care for us, really. You have to have grown up in a normal family, or read about how to do it somewhere, but she didn't know."

It's surprising, this glimpse of a past version of my mother, a version who understood why my grandmother did the things she did, or tried to, and was able to forgive her.

I reread the autopsy report she sent me, years before, when she started investigating her father's death. It tells me my grandfather was six feet tall and very thin and that he served in the army reserves. That he was found by a teenage employee completely naked and dead underneath the Cadillac Seville whose engine he was working on. That his last known location alive was at the home of a white woman, a woman who was not his wife. And I understand the appeal the mystery of his death held for my mother, how the answer became for a while the door through which she thought she might walk and emerge from the prison created by the question of his loss.

IN HOUSTON, REESE AND I interviewed climate experts at Rice University who broke down for us how the modern concept of "the good life" was built entirely on the idea of almost free, unlimited oil. Oil, they said, was the beating heart of Houston, the nation's metabolic force. It pumped its way out of Louisiana, Texas, and Oklahoma and breathed life into the rest of the country. The American Dream was the dream of Houston, of unlimited fuel.

Now, back in the rehearsal room in Irvine, the music turns mournful as the movement moves toward its end. The choir sings lines from oral histories gathered from workers on the rigs:

We thought the Gulf would heal itself.
We thought it would never end.

The utter destruction of the Gulf Coast. The rise of a radical right funded by conservative billionaires. A politics that normalizes war for oil. The world we live in is haunted by all the other ones that were and might have been. This piece is meant to be an accounting of their ghosts. But how can I complete it honestly if I won't also account for the ghosts that haunt me?

...

MY AGENT PLACES A STORY I wrote, about a girl who goes on a trip to Baja with her rich white boyfriend and embarrasses herself by feeding tacos to the stray village dogs, in a national magazine. I'm invited to the issue launch party at a hotel in downtown Los Angeles. I'm intimidated by the magazine's cultural cachet, but Sadie has plans to be in town the same weekend and agrees to come with me as my plus-one. As I step into the hotel foyer, I'm greeted by the associate editor, who has pale skin; long, dark hair; and bright blue eyes. I give her my name.

"Oh, it's you! I loved your story," she says.

"Thank you. I love the magazine," I answer, beaming. Is it my imagination, or does her smile fade and then return, less genuine than before? Have I broken yet another unspoken, unknowable rule? This is how it always is for me at these events: Am I being laughed at? Do I sound stupid? Does the person I'm talking to wish they were talking to someone better? But then I spot Sadie stationed in front of a booth giving out free samples of Japanese whiskey. For ten years, I have been searching for Sadie in crowded rooms full of strangers and, when I find her, letting out a breath I didn't know I was holding.

I drain the glass she hands me and relax into the melty feeling of the party. Sadie tells me an old teacher reached out to ask for an introduction to Sadie's agent, a very big name in the industry. "Can you believe that?" Sadie says, offended. "I haven't talked to this woman in years."

I clink her glass with mine, happy now that I know what kind of night it will be, a night for shit-talking. I tell her about an old coworker who keeps using our past conversations as content for her job writing Buzzfeed lists. Actual conversations about '90s heart-throbs and unconventional personality traits repurposed as the inescapable headlines I'm always having to scroll past on my phone. It wouldn't matter so much if this person hadn't abruptly stopped speaking to me. We were friends and then I left for New York, and when I came back we were not friends anymore.

"If anybody did something like that to me, I would punch them in the face," Sadie says, and she is serious, unequivocal. I appreciate her saying this, for making it okay for me to think it without guilt. I drink another cocktail and take a butterscotch budino off a passing tray. Anthony Bourdain walks in, causing a stir. Sadie excuses herself to go ask for a photo. At the same time, two authors I'm friendly with, Kate Yoon and Eliza Schiff, arrive. When Sadie comes back, I introduce them. The conversation turns to the 2016 presidential election. "Hillary only became the Democratic nominee because she's married to Bill," Sadie, a staunch Bernie Sanders supporter, says in response to something I didn't hear.

"That's not true," Kate says. "She and Bill were classmates at Yale. He was president when she couldn't have been. He's not why she's powerful." Then Kate reels off a list of Hillary's qualifications. She was a senator. She worked on the Watergate commission. She was an outspoken feminist and one of the only female law professors at the university where she taught.

Sadie's eyes go wide. Her breath hitches. She likes being lectured almost as much as she likes being argued with—which is to say not at all. Sadie expects deference, and when she doesn't get it, does not bother to hide how this disrespect makes her feel.

"I'm sorry, but did I do something to you?" Kate answers, finally registering Sadie's disdain, her voice now cold. At this point I remember feeling surprised, and maybe even a little glad, that Kate, who was not afraid of conflict, was responding to Sadie's rudeness in kind. Sadie was my best friend but she was also often curt with me, and I hadn't known retaliation of any sort was allowed.

"Why?" Sadie asks just as icily.

"You're staring at me really angrily," Kate says, her voice now aggressively neutral.

"Oh, so now I'm angry?" Sadie says. Her own tone is brittle. There is nothing neutral about it. Everyone within hearing distance has fallen silent.

Eliza tries to change the subject to a recent local housing bill. Sadie, rigid with frustration, turns abruptly, headed in the direction of the elevator that will take her down to the street. I chase her, already feeling guilty and acutely aware that, though Kate incited her indignation, I invited her to this party and so it is my job to fix it.

"Are you okay?" I ask as I catch up to her.

Sadie looks at me in stunned disbelief. "That girl called me angry."

It's clear what she's insinuating and I want to be a loyal friend, but I'm finding it difficult. Kate called Sadie angry. The angry Black woman is an insidious stereotype. But it's also accurate to say that Sadie is angry at Kate.

"Kate's not racist," I say, because she isn't, and you can't make lies up about people who don't deserve it because they disagree with you. It's not fighting fair.

Sadie laughs darkly. "Okay," she says. She looks at me with a mixture of pity and contempt I recognize from my mother's face.

What I want to say to her, but don't: *Why are you acting like this?*

What I imagine she wants to say back to me: Why aren't *you?*

LATER THAT WEEKEND, I LISTEN to an interview Sadie did with a well-known literary podcast in which she is brash and a little mean to the host, compelling him to impress her rather than the other way around, which he seems eager to do. I wonder again if her approach—anger all the time as opposed to emotional deadness—might be healthier than mine.

"Assholes usually win," Ethan agrees, when I present my theory to him that night in more general terms. "That's true. People don't trust nice."

"Does that mean I should be an asshole?"

"I'm not going to dignify that with a response," Ethan says.

"No, seriously. How can I become an asshole?"

"It's not something you become," he says, exasperated. "It's something you are."

"So I'm stuck? I have to be a nice loser?"

"It's not—" Ethan considers. "Sadie is not an asshole to other people. She's an asshole with her time. Assholes only respond to what they want to respond to in ways that will help them. That's a big part of why she's so successful. You let everybody in."

Ethan doesn't know about the fight at the party. I haven't told him. I'm not sure how to think about what happened. I'm confused, actually. I still don't know which one of us was right. "To be a Negro in this country and to be relatively conscious is to be in a state of rage almost, almost all of the time," said James Baldwin.[21] Maybe my problem is I don't know what righteous anger is supposed to look like. Maybe I conflate it too easily with my mother's anger and my own fear of being consumed by it. Of losing my mind.

I look up the phrase "Black psychosis" and learn, or relearn, the word "drapetomania." Coined by a Virginia doctor and slaveholder named Samuel Cartwright, it denotes a madness attributed to Black enslaved men and women intent on running away from the white people who owned them.[22] Cartwright also invented the term "dysaesthesia aethiopica," defined as a form of madness manifesting as "rascality" and "disrespect for the master's property." The cure for both disorders was "extensive whipping."

I learn early American psychiatrists suggested Black people lacked the capacity for freedom, and thought this lack led to a rise in insanity cases after slavery was abolished. "A crazy Negro was a rare sight before emancipation. . . . We know he is by no means rare today," wrote psychiatrist Arrah Evarts in 1914.[23] Her detailed case studies of freed slaves feature patients who beat their heads against walls, sang hymns, and repeated verses from the Bible.

But I also learn that in 1927, E. Franklin Frazier, the first Black head of the American Sociological Society, published an essay entitled "The Pathology of Race Prejudice," arguing that white people's "social incapacity" when it comes to Black people is itself a form of insanity. He writes, "Southern white people afflicted with the Negro-complex show themselves incapable of performing certain social functions."[24] The very claim to "understand" the Negro, he asserts, points to a sick mind incapable of grasping new information.

Finally, I learn that in a late essay on psychosis, Freud noted that "mankind as a whole," like the schizophrenia patient, ". . . has developed delusions which are inaccessible to logical criticism and which contradict reality."[25]

LATER, I WATCH A VIDEO my grandmother sends of the rooms of her chiropractic office filling up with junk. "DON'T LISTEN TO LANCE BLANKS. HE'S ONLY TRYING TO HURT YOU," is scrawled in Sharpie across one wall. I see the dark impression of a foot in the floorboards, and though I will eventually learn that this is the result of wood rot, at the time, it looks like my mother lit the floor on fire and then stepped into the flames.

"You know your mother," my grandmother says with a sigh when I call her. "She can be kind of hardheaded. She needs to learn you can't go through life on autopilot. She'll make the changes she needs to make."

"Right," I say. "But it doesn't sound like she's in a state to even think like that?"

"Well, she's not getting along with the people at her church anymore. She said some woman followed her. Of course, that was during an episode, but women can be catty. Anyway, she quit going to her regular church, and now she's going to the homeless church."

"The homeless church?"

"It's a church for homeless people. One of my patients goes there—he's been diagnosed with schizophrenia—and he has a group down there he never misses. Says he gets a lot out of it."

"She needs to keep going. Can you make her do that?"

"Sure. I can drive her over there," my grandmother says, a little dismissive. "I bought her some books on personal improvement." It's as if she believes as long as she doesn't address my mother's diagnosis, it can't hurt us and it won't be real. Is this, I wonder, an example of one of Freud's delusions which is inaccessible to logical criticism and contradicts reality?

I hang up and call my mother.

"HELLO," she says.

"Mom?" A long silence follows. "Hello? Are you okay?"

"Oh, I'm alright. You have to talk real loud! I can't hear you over all these cars."

She is shouting. I'm immediately alert. "Where are you?"

"I'm walking down C. E. King Parkway." I hear barking. "Listen, I have to go. There are these—um, dogs? I have some spray."

"Hello? Mom?" But she's no longer on the other end of the line. I call back and she doesn't answer. I look up C. E. King Parkway on Google Maps. Houston is not a city where anyone walks. This highway, in particular, does not look suitable for pedestrians. I call again and then again, but she doesn't pick up. I wait in a state of high anxiety until later that evening when Aunt Tina texts to tell me my mother has been home for hours.

...

THE CALIFORNIA CHORUS holds a press conference to announce their new season. Reese and I meet in a well-appointed lounge on the second floor of Disney Hall to present our oratorio to the assembled reporters. The luxurious setting, the journalists, the table of hors d'oeuvres laid out at the bar all look the way I imagined success would look, but somehow I don't feel like I'm there. It's as if what's happening is happening to somebody else.

I tell the reporters about the libretto's first movement, about the life of Robert Church, whose mother was a slave and whose father owned riverboats that ran up and down the Mississippi. When slavery ended and Church was freed, he started his own riverboat business, which expanded to billiard halls and brothels. He became the first black millionaire in Tennessee. He bought a house with over a dozen rooms, where he hosted Frederick Douglass and Booker T. Washington and agitated for the Black vote. During Jim Crow, when Black people were kept out of white establishments, he opened a Black public park, an auditorium, and a bank. Church's son, Robert Church Jr., went to Oberlin and worked on Wall Street, then took over the bank his father ran before entering politics. His granddaughter, Roberta Church, was the first Black woman in Memphis to be elected to public office.

AFTER I INTRODUCE THE LIBRETTO, Reese discusses the music, and then the tall, thin, elegant man who commissioned our piece and who conducts the choir and whom it is impossible to imagine working any job other than classical music conductor stands up to talk to the gathered crowd. "This piece," he says, "carries a message of such great hope."

But that's not true. What we're after is more nuanced than that, darker. We are looking at the moment before the moment everything changes and then changes again. The point at which a new world looks possible but before it has arrived. Not hope, but thresholds and what crossing them costs.

Researching Robert Church, we learned the Memphis Housing Authority authorized the Church house to be burned down in 1953 to test new fire equipment. This was after the city had seized the house from the family for delinquent taxes and refused to allow Robert Church Jr. to pay them.[26] More recently, the city built a housing project specifically for Black people on top of the land where the house once stood. The previous year, we'd flown to Memphis to see these projects, brightly painted A-frame structures behind iron gates already falling into disrepair. I remember watching a child alone on a porch swing a dirty stuffed rabbit in circles by its ear. I thought of the house my grandmother bought us in Riverside Terrace, a different kind of memorial to another hoped-for upward trajectory that didn't pan out, and I wanted to fight somebody.

WHEN I ASK MY GRANDMOTHER to tell me more about my grandfather she writes me back emails full of unadorned anecdotes that read as if she's writing about somebody else. She tells me that during an argument, he grabbed her by the hair and threw her against the wall so hard he sent her to the emergency room. When he dropped her off at work the following Monday, she called her brother to help her pick up my mother and Aunt Tina from day care, got her things from home, and moved in with a cousin.

My grandfather, who didn't want a divorce, made my grandmother's life hell, transferring his assets to his brother to avoid paying child support, breaking into her new house and ransacking it, stalking her through the city. My great-grandmother Alma came to Houston to help her daughter move, and one day Vernon followed them into a parking lot, threatening to take the children. Alma brandished a steak knife she'd been keeping in her purse for just this purpose. He filed charges against Alma, and she did a short stay in jail.

Now I think it must have come as a shock to my grandmother that Alma protected her, given that, as she explained, Alma never seemed to like her very much. My great-grandmother favored her two sons over her only daughter and generally only addressed my grandmother to scold or threaten her.

It startles me to realize how much my grandmother's mother resembles my own mother in her ferocity and sadness. My mother is repeating her own trauma in me, but Alma is inside her too. Alma's mother, my great-great-grandmother Sarah, was the daughter of an enslaved woman from Georgia and the son of the white man who purchased her at auction. So what unknown history was Alma repeating?

AFTER WE WENT TO SEE the former site of the Church house in Memphis, I went by myself to the National Civil Rights Museum at the Lorraine Motel to see an exhibit on the Atlantic slave trade. I walked past a life-sized cross-section of a slave ship hold with people in it packed back to chest, a replica of a woman on an auction block holding a baby while a slaver called for bids, an enslaved couple attempting to run with their baby, their faces twisted with fear.

I know from my grandmother's research that Charity Rice, my grandmother's great-grandmother, sailed into Galveston and was auctioned off to a slaveholder in Nacogdoches. She became a "mistress" to the slaveholder's son, and they were listed in the 1880 census as living together. They had four children, of whom Sarah (my grandmother's grandmother) was the youngest. Before Charity, my grandmother says, the names stop.

At the museum, I listened to oral histories of the Montgomery bus boycott. I saw the room in the Lorraine Motel where Martin Luther King Jr. slept the night before he was murdered, staged behind glass so the sheets were still messy, as if he'd recently left. I called a rideshare to take me back to my rental, and on the way home I asked the driver if he'd grown up in Memphis and whether he liked it here. He complained about the high murder rates, which were, he said, due largely to "Black-on-Black crime."

I gestured out the window at the boarded-up storefronts and empty, overgrown plots of land we were passing. I told him about how agents of corrupt Memphis leadership chased business-owning blacks out of town and set their property on fire. What had been done to the Black community in Memphis was done intentionally, and there were repercussions for everyone, as he could see. He drove the rest of the way in silence. After he dropped me off, I tried to send him a list of books to read, but I kept messing up the allowable character count, and the message I sent ultimately was unhinged.

On the plane home to Los Angeles, I watched the 2016 election returns. I thought the reality in the plane must have been different, that they must have been running the wrong tape and, once

I landed, everything would be in order again. It was only when I made it back to my apartment to find Ethan watching CNN that I understood we were entering a new world that was, at the same time, only the old world on repeat. Everything that was going to happen had happened already, before, and would continue to happen again.

BACK IN LOS ANGELES, SADIE calls to see if I want to come visit the Airbnb where she's staying while she's in town for a book festival. I arrive carrying a tub of hummus and a box of crackers and tell her the latest about my mother, how she won't take medication and we don't know what to do. The strangest thing about schizophrenia, I tell her as I set out snacks for us, is that it's not terminal but it's also not treatable without meds. She won't die. She'll only get worse, forever.

"Listen," Sadie says, with an abruptness that startles me, "it's not your job to save your mom." And, while she's right, it doesn't matter.

We gossip about writers she's run into on tour—which ones are overrated, which ones aren't getting the attention they deserve—and I congratulate her on having been shortlisted for a major award. I tell her about the notes on my novel, my agent saying the graduate student, Mark, is too hard to envision, that I need to make him more clearly visible and less vague. Why does Laura feel anything for Mark, she keeps asking? Why does she care so much about finding Canton's book?

We're interrupted by the arrival of Sadie's friend Emma, a translator and the girlfriend of an editor we both know named Phillip. Sadie pours us each a glass of expensive sipping tequila sent to her by her editor and soon we are pleasantly drunk. Conversation turns to the next Democratic primary. She brings up Bernie Sanders, on whose campaign she hopes to work in some capacity when he becomes the 2020 Democratic Presidential nominee. I wonder out loud if the nomination might be out of reach because he is so polarizing.

"But he's the most popular politician in the United States right now," Sadie says. She sounds offended on his behalf, as if she is his friend.

"Look at how defensive you get at the mention of his name," I shoot back. "That's exactly my point."

She aims a glare at me so dirty that for a moment, I think she's going to spit. A gap appears between us that no one else can see.

Emma breaks the tension by bringing up writers we all know who live on the East Coast. Next year, she's starting a research fellowship at the New York Public Library. Then Sadie changes the subject to a video she recently texted me that she took on her phone. In it, a white woman in a parking lot outside Target appeals to a security guard offscreen for help. Offscreen, Sadie demands the woman "tell them what you did!" The woman tells the security guard Sadie is following her and she is scared. The security guard, looking bewildered, tells Sadie she's not allowed to film inside the store without permission. The video cuts off.

The white woman spoke to Sadie rudely in the parking lot for not returning her cart to the drop-off, so Sadie followed her inside. She replays the scene for Emma and me in the suite kitchen.

"You about to be a social media star, bitch!" she shouts, waving her phone around. I feel a gnawing in my stomach the way I do when I am talking to my mother and it becomes apparent she is operating according to rules of a world I'm not in.

"What a bitch," I say back to Sadie half-heartedly about the white woman.

Sadie's New Year's resolution is to not take any shit, she says. She's calling out all the assholes. I tell her she should run for office, and she says she's thinking about it.

After Emma leaves, Sadie offers to help me spread the word about the upcoming premiere of my oratorio. She has access to a list of media contacts she's happy to share. I say sure and give her a hug before I leave, but on the ride home I feel distinctly terrible.

A KEY CONFLICT AT THE heart of Walter Benjamin's relationship with his closest friend, the scholar Gershom Scholem, was Benjamin's Jewishness.[27] Scholem thought Judaism didn't figure enough into Benjamin's intellectual life and disapproved of how much of his philosophy existed outside it. At one point he offered the perennially broke Benjamin a position as an instructor at Hebrew University, where Scholem taught, if only Benjamin would take Hebrew lessons, which the university would cover. Benjamin accepted the money but never took the lessons and later had to admit to Scholem that he had no true interest in Judaism except inasmuch as he was interested in Scholem.

When I learned about this, I thought of Sadie, who writes about Blackness unabashedly and who has made fun of me, in the past, for being "postracial." I'm not postracial, but a Blackness that de-fines itself entirely oppositionally is never a type of Black I learned how to be. Before I met Sadie, I didn't know how to talk about my relationship to identity without feeling weird, but she'd also gone to mostly white schools and she understood what it meant to live in the in-between. This was, at one time, a topic we discussed a lot, but now it's become another thing we don't talk about, the same way we don't talk about the tacit but obvious pressure for Black authors to write and speak a certain way, or my fear that Sadie has given in to that pressure uncritically in exchange for her book's success and that doing so may have detrimental downstream ef-fects. Her success in general is another thing we don't talk about, just as we don't talk about my envy of it and, thus far, my failure.

REFLECTING ON HIS FRIENDSHIP WITH Benjamin, Scholem writes, "There were many things that Benjamin, being the way he was, could not express in letters—and this became increasingly true as the years advanced. This meant that we sought no con-flict but also that the things we avoided were magnified by silence. Thus too many of the things that ought to have achieved a thor-ough clarification in a discussion between two friends remained in abeyance. The ensuing five years suffered from this. Something had remained mute that had not been designed to be so, and like everything thus unspoken, it was dangerous."[28]

EIGHT

I START A SUMMER JOB teaching middle and high school students creative writing at an arts camp in Virginia. On the first day, I bring in an Amy Hempel short story, "The Man in Bogotá," in which a narrator watches a TV news story about a suicidal woman poised on a ledge and is reminded of a different story about an industrialist who was kidnapped and held for ransom. His kidnappers forced him to give up smoking and to exercise and eat better so he would survive until the money came together, and when he was released, his doctor told him that the kidnapping was "the best thing to happen" to him. It ends with the narrator recounting the tale of the industrialist to the woman on the ledge. The narrator thinks, "Maybe this is not a come-down-from-the-ledge story. But I tell it with the thought that the woman on the ledge will ask herself a question, the question that occurred to that man in Bogotá. He wondered how we know that what happens to us isn't good."[29]

After we read it, the students blink at me in their kind, optimistic, intelligent way, waiting for me to explain what Hempel means here. But I have not prepared an explanation.

On another day, I pass out writing prompts consisting of excerpts from Kafka that I like—"No psychology ever again!" he proclaims on one otherwise entirely blank page of *The Zürau*

Aphorisms[30]—and a few students look at me with concern. When I get my evaluations back halfway through the course, one student has written *Sometimes the class feels a little bit serious. I know we're in class and all; it just seems a little extreme sometimes.*

Still, all summer, the kids do things that make my heart jump into my throat. During a sudden storm, they all rise from their seats and rush as one to the window to watch sheets of rain fall from the black sky. On talent night, a girl plays a song she wrote on the guitar. She looks like the child Ethan and I might have, with skin and hair the color and texture at the exact point where mine and Ethan's meet. And I think if I do have a child, and that kid can write songs and sing them, then taking the risk of becoming my mother by becoming a mother myself might be worth it.

To have children and not be prepared for the possibility of schizophrenia would be irresponsible. But that's not a reason not to have them if I want them. What if my grandmother had opted not to have my mother? What if my mother had opted not to have me? You become a mother and that's who you are, my mother used to say to me. Would she have been better off if she hadn't become a mother? If not, who would she have become?

In *The Arcades Project*, Benjamin includes this passage written by Claire Démar, an obscure nineteenth-century writer and member of the avant-garde:

No more motherhood! No more law of the blood. I say: no more motherhood. And, in fact, the woman emancipated . . . from the man, who then no longer pays her the price of her body . . . will owe her existence . . . to her works alone.[31]

I tend to agree. But then there is also the fact that Démar killed herself at the age of thirty-four. I wonder if it was worth it to her to live thirty-four years of a life that owed its existence to her works alone. Sometimes I think for me it might be. That if I could write one perfect novel, I would never ask the universe for anything else, and would be fine with dying immediately after. Other times, that line of thought feels unhinged. Plenty of people who don't write novels lead wonderful lives, and plenty of people who do write novels are miserable. In fact, there appears to be an inverse correlation between writing good novels and having a good life. Meanwhile, most of the people I know who have children don't talk to me about whether or not they are happy. They talk about their children and how much they love them and how well or badly they have taken to potty-training. For this reason, having children also feels to me like a kind of death, only on the other side you come out not as a corpse but as someone whose happiness depends upon the toilet habits of a human you yourself created and set upon the world. Which is not a bad thing. Which, might in fact, be a sort of solution.

In *The Fire Next Time*, James Baldwin writes:

Perhaps the whole root of our trouble, the human trouble, is that we will sacrifice all the beauty of our lives, will imprison ourselves in totems, taboos, crosses, blood sacrifices, steeples, mosques, races, armies, flags, nations, in order to deny the fact of death, which is the only fact we have. It seems to me that one ought to rejoice in the *fact* of death—ought to decide, indeed, to *earn* one's death by confronting with passion the conundrum of life.[32]

Which actually, in the end, is no help at all, given that he does not name the tenets of this conundrum.

FOR THE LOS ANGELES MOVEMENT of our oratorio, Morgan has set up an interview at the Jet Propulsion Laboratory. The scientist we meet, Adam Steltzner, has been profiled in *The New Yorker*, which impresses me more than it should and more than the fact that he is the chief engineer for the next major expedition to the surface of Mars. He works out of a smallish corner office with a window overlooking the JPL campus, equations scattered over a whiteboard on the opposite wall. He's tall with a pouf of curled hair that makes him look like Elvis. He used to be in a band, and the first thing he does is show us a photo of himself as a younger man, on a record cover.

I tell him we are there to interview him about the role of Los Angeles in humanity's expansion into space. He thinks for a second, then tells us that he's devoted his life and career to finding out whether Mars was ever alive or if it could be, but that Mars itself is not the point and neither are these questions. The point is the exploration. The esoteric, impractical nature of it. The ideas within the search that allow us to look for and find the edge of what people are capable of.

People have been asking questions about the limits of human potential since before we learned to make fire, he says, when we could only find it burning already, mostly from lightning strikes. We used it to light other fires but couldn't keep it. He tells us these fires were an unusual opportunity for humans to see time: wood becoming ash in front of our eyes slowly, always changing. That awareness of time allowed for meditative contemplation, and it was in these periods that humans learned how to plan for the future.

"We must understand," he says emphatically, "that the idea that we represent the pinnacle of life in this universe is terrifying. We careen all over the place. We're too unpredictable. If we're it for life in the universe, well, that's too depressing an idea to contemplate."

But I don't find this idea depressing at all. Vast near-infinite years of nothingness, then microwave background radiation, then gas giants, stars, planets, then people. Human beings are only a function of probability, proof anything warm eventually turns into something else, even almost empty space. Anything could have happened, and humans were what did. If that was all we got in this lifetime for meaning, why couldn't it be enough?

And what has ambition gotten anybody, ever? I think later at my desk, sifting through my notes from the interview. My grandmother was ambitious, and now she's stuck taking care of a psychotic daughter she won't admit is psychotic and who doesn't want to be taken care of. I was ambitious, and my chosen field barely exists anymore, literary fiction and criticism all churned into the maw of an internet that cannot find a way to commoditize them and so has set about eradicating them under the guise of their being elitist and boring, which they mostly are.

Ethan looked shocked the first time I couldn't come to bed right away because I said I had to write, back when I was still stupid enough to think writing every day was how I was going to become a writer. "Write what?" he said, and I said, "I don't know, thoughts from my day?" I let him read some of the journal I was keeping then in a document several hundred pages long, and he looked at it and then looked at me and said, "You don't miss anything, do you?"

I felt flattered. His was the exact response I'd been looking for. But now the words ring out like an accusation. How can I live my life if I am only ever standing apart from it? Watching it? What do I think I'm doing? In trying to write about the connections between layered realities, I erased all my connections to this one. I thought to get to where I wanted to be I had to separate myself from the world, but now I don't know how to get back. The support group for people with mentally ill loved ones that I attend regularly now is the first sustained amount of time I've spent with a group of people outside of work since graduate school.

I change into jogging clothes, step outside as the last lick of daylight dissolves, and run uphill into the night. I've been running the same route in my neighborhood for so long that I've watched the bright-eyed, dark-haired children of Los Feliz grow taller through the window of the violin teacher on Rowena, watched the Lab puppy on St. George grow fat and slow and gray, watched his elderly Boston terrier friend disappear. And because so little about my life has changed, it sometimes feels as if all this time passed over the course of a day, or an hour, rather than half a decade.

What scares me most is my mother didn't know where her turning point was. It came and went without announcing itself, and by the time we recognized it, it was too late. I ran away from home so the moment wouldn't find me, but in doing so, I wonder now if I've only ensured it will.

NINE

MY MOTHER'S MESSAGES FILL UP my phone like dark poems.

Sarah, can you come to Houston? Lance keeps saying you're dead from cyanide poisoning.

He scares me. He makes me think you are not you. I'm sorry.

Lance is saying he did something to my phone so I can't receive texts from you.

Please call me.

please go to the police

I send her a text telling her to ignore Lance because he is only trying to hurt her. I call Ethan in Guatemala, where he is teaching a film class, to tell him I've had an epiphany. It doesn't matter to me whether we get married or not. Marriage is a top-down imposition and therefore doomed to failure. Love is supposed to bloom organically. I like how we choose each other every day. Marriage, I say, would ruin everything.

"What?" he says. He sounds irritated. "I don't see why you have to be such a downer all the time. You're putting a damper on a surprise."

Is the surprise a ring? I ask. Does it have a blood diamond in it? Do jewelry stores still carry blood diamonds? And if it's not a blood diamond, if it's whatever the opposite of a blood diamond is, what will happen when I inevitably lose it? The way I have lost every other valuable object anyone has ever given me? And now I am crying and saying things that don't quite make sense. The money Ethan would spend on a ring could go toward a new apartment, I say, or another dog for Larry Bird to play with. She is such a good dog, and all she wants to do is run around outside, but we don't have a yard, and the security guard at the park keeps threatening to give us tickets for letting her off-leash when she is not supposed to be off-leash and—

"You don't have to have a ring if you don't want to," Ethan says.

No, I tell him, I definitely want a ring. The need for him to buy me a diamond feels primal. That's what I want, more than anything, for Ethan to go spelunking and to bring me back a wild diamond so big it proves he's capable of providing for the children I'm afraid to have.

REESE AND I MEET WITH a man named Richard Dayton. He works for a tech company based in Los Angeles that is offering a thirty-million-dollar award for the first privately funded teams to land a rocket on the moon.

"We're trying to make it possible for private companies to explore space," he tells us when we visit him in an office park on the west side. "Just like the early days of American colonization."

He tells us there are shadowed craters on the moon's north and south poles where there are thought to exist large amounts of ice. He thinks we might someday establish lunar bases where the soil of the moon—the rigoleth—can be mined for water.

"So you'll have these fascinating mining operations there in extremely cold temperatures just below you," he explains, "and you'd be situated on this higher point where you will have eternal light."

Richard thinks it's a basic attribute of our species that we want to explore new horizons. There was a time, he reminds us, when people in western Europe didn't know about the continent of America. And when they first found America, they weren't even looking for America, he explains, they were looking for the Indies.

"What happened after they found America?" Reese asks him dryly.

"Well, look," Richard says. He glances at me. He swallows. "There might be conflict. All the things we've done in the past are likely to show up in one way or another. But we won't need slavery, because we would have robots. And not just anybody would get to go. These people would be . . . selected."

"Selected how?" I ask.

"Highly educated. Ready to set a good example for the rest of humanity," Richard answers. There will be crime, he admits. Maybe war. Maybe diseases and pests. But those are simply imperfections that humanity takes with us everywhere we go.

Nevertheless, he insists, within a hundred years we'll be living across the solar system. We'll visit the asteroids. We'll go to Mars's two moons. We'll land on the surface of Mars itself, and there we will, perhaps, find a new home.

THREE WEEKS LATER, I VISIT Ethan in a vacation village in Guatemala called Antigua. We hike the side of a volcano with our friend Jorge, who works at the university with Ethan. Near the peak, Jorge

NO ONE GETS TO FALL APART

lags behind, while Ethan leads me to a slightly higher peak. He proposes with a ring hidden inside a copy of *War and Peace*, on the title page of which he has inscribed the poem "Corazón coraza," by Mario Benedetti. When I say yes, Ethan says, "Really?" as if he's shocked, which I understand completely. Because we are on the side of an active volcano, the two-minute video Jorge shoots of the proposal looks like a scene from a Tarkovsky film, smoky gray light over black rock, clouds moving in as we kiss.

In the dark of Jorge's family guesthouse, where we are staying, I think about my mother, wonder if she ever got proposed to, if she ever said to herself, *Now I am engaged.* The ring makes my finger look different, expensive, as if the hand it belongs to deserves to be treated with care. Some part of me wants to cut it off and mount it on the wall.

Later, Ethan's colleague brings us a bottle of champagne and we toast. Aunt Tina, whom Ethan alerted before the proposal and who used two of her vacation passes at the airline so she and my grandmother could come with us on this trip, is thrilled. But my grandmother, who didn't know, and who distrusts the entire institution of marriage, says, "I don't understand why you two would do that. When everything was going so well."

ANTIGUA WAS DESTROYED BY AN earthquake in 1773, and the new city sprouting out of the ruins of the old one forms a kind of palimpsest. Half-collapsed churches and monasteries sit everywhere, vines and grasses draped over their roofs and growing up between the broken walls of the colonial buildings. A centuries-old convent, Casa Santo Domingo, has been redeveloped into an upscale hotel with a Sunday buffet. We go there for a celebratory brunch. During our meal, I check my phone and immediately wish I hadn't. My mother has called me three times. My grandmother looks at her own phone and then gets up and leaves the table. I follow her to the bathroom, where I find her talking to a cop back in the States.

My mother, left behind in Houston, went to my grandmother's condo, couldn't find her there, and now believes she is missing, and so she has called the police. My grandmother speaks politely to the officer and explains that she is on vacation. My mother calls me again, and I don't answer the phone. My grandmother returns to the table and explains why she hadn't mentioned anything to my mother about leaving Houston: my mother has taken to spending the night with a homeless man, and my grandmother didn't want her to bring him back to the office. My mother had gifted the man some of my grandmother's things, including a tent and a set of beloved ikat-patterned luggage. She said he was the only person she had to talk to.

My grandmother quietly informs Aunt Tina about the situation. Meanwhile, we're joined for brunch by the white-haired, blue-eyed director of development for the university where Ethan teaches. I've told the woman about my novel, and she wants to tell me about a radio interview she heard in which a scientist suggested what we think of as supernatural occurrences might actually be proof our universe is only one of many. She looked for the interview online but never found it again—which, she tells me, seems like a supernatural occurrence in itself. It's hard to pay attention to what she is saying, because my aunt and my grandmother keep whispering to each other about my mother across the table. I am terrified something else is going to happen to her while we are here. Something worse. Aunt Tina senses my anxiety and asks why I'm not talking.

"Don't worry about her," she tells me. "She'll be fine."

Define "fine," I want to say, but don't.

Ethan stays in Guatemala to finish out the semester, and I return to our apartment in Los Angeles. All day, my phone vibrates with texts.

Lance is crazy Sarah

He is threatening you with harassment right now

I am asking you to go file a restraining order

Please go to the police. Please go see if you can file a restraining order

He is saying he is going to kill you

I send a message back reassuring her I'm safe. I talk to the dog for long stretches at a time as the apartment decorates itself with copies of the Sunday New York Times, delivered to our front porch, brought in but never opened because the subscription is Ethan's and he is not here to open them. I watch my bank account deplete as the fridge fills with takeout spring rolls and half-empty containers of curry. When I eat food and don't give any to the dog, she stares at me until I relent. "Are you my love?" I say. I'm lying down on the floor, facing her, looking into her eyes. She blinks at me and licks my nose. I wonder where my mother would be now if she liked animals. If a cat or a fish or a bird could have saved her.

MY MOTHER IS PICKED UP by the cops and hospitalized again. She checks herself out and breaks a window in my grandmother's office to let herself in. She denies breaking the window when confronted about it. "If she's not willing to see the doctor or something, she's going to have to apply for food stamps. It doesn't make sense for me to have to support a fifty-two-year-old woman," my grandmother says when I call.

"Do you want me to come back again?" I ask.

Instead of answering, she sighs. "They're posting about her online."

I open the Nextdoor app on my phone, plug in my grandmother's zip code, and discover she is right. One person from the area is complaining about the notes my mother is leaving in his mailbox. Someone else accuses her of tossing a jar of pee at their house. A sympathetic neighbor named Rachel, who is white, writes: Please know that she is a mentally ill resident of our neighborhood and not a transient. We are very much hoping that she will not do anything out of line again ☺

THEN AUNT TINA TEXTS WITH good news: she's cajoled my mother into joining a free community treatment program in Houston. She'll have access to free medication management, group therapy, and counseling, all provided by the state.

Aunt Tina went with her to her first psychiatry appointment and it went relatively well. When the psychiatrist asked my mother who helps her, my aunt reports, she named Hakeem Olajuwon, a Hall of Fame NBA basketball star who played center for the Houston Rockets in the '90s. Not Aunt Tina, who brings her meals every day, or my grandmother, who pays for my mother to live.

My aunt seems tickled by this, not peeved. A young social worker, Courtney, has already visited her twice to make sure she's taking her antipsychotics. My aunt likes Courtney, tells me she's sweet. And already my mother appears to be getting better. She's not shouting as much or throwing things or destroying my grandmother's possessions.

I ask for the social worker's number and leave her a message with some follow-up questions. When she finally calls me back, I realize she'd already returned my call, days before, and that I didn't pick up because I thought her call was spam. That was on a Thursday. It's now Sunday. How many things is it possible for me to do wrong?

I text the social worker all the information I have about my mother. I ask her for the psychiatrist's contact information and she shares it, but the psychiatrist won't speak to me. Says it would be a violation of confidentiality rules. In fact, Courtney tells me, she got in trouble for giving me his number. It's clear Courtney would like me to stop texting her. But I don't, so she stops responding.

Alone in Los Feliz, I wrap my arms around my knees. Depression unfurls like a black cloth. I imagine lying down in the street outside my apartment. Banging my head against my car window until it breaks. Renting a room with my savings and letting my body be discovered by the smell. At night, I pray for earthquakes, car accidents, drowning, anything that might offer reprieve. I don't know how to help my mother—the same way I don't know how to fight a disease that means always trying to outrun yourself.

TEN

IN NOVEMBER 2017 I TAKE a cheap flight to New York to do a reading at the Poetry Project for the launch of a literary journal called *Encyclopedia* that is publishing a short story I wrote about my mother's quest for the truth about her father's death. In the city, I have drinks with Jill and we talk about the latest draft of my novel—she can see how much work I've done, she says, though the way she says it isn't very convincing. Before I can push, though, we've switched topics to the #MeToo wave that is sweeping up so many powerful men in its path. The month before, in October, sexual assault allegations against the film producer Harvey Weinstein bubbled up to the surface of public consciousness and set off a wave of reckonings. Story after story poured forth. As of this morning, a famous white female director and outspoken feminist has found herself in the crosshairs of the movement. She defended a white TV writer, a friend of hers, who was accused of raping a young Black actress. In defending the writer, she suggested the actress was lying about having been raped. Her fans and followers are enraged at her hypocrisy.

We talk about this story and about #MeToo as a whole. Jill knows someone impacted by the movement. I know someone. We don't know what's happening, but we know the balance of power is shifting and the shift has to do with race, with power, with beauty, with class. We change the subject. My novel is getting there, she assures me. But the relationship at its heart, between Mark and Laura, still isn't working, and maybe the issue that needs to be driven home harder is less one of time travel and romance, in fact, more one of race.

"You do see what I'm saying?" she asks me finally, both of us a little embarrassed for each other and for ourselves. "About the love story not working?"

I do. The love story isn't working because I still have not managed to make Mark, the graduate student, feel three-dimensional, and now I'm stuck with him at the center of my story, where he takes up all the oxygen without producing any forward motion. I hate this character because his unreality pervades the entire manuscript, infecting all its other parts. I can't remove him from the book, because if I do, the whole creaky foundation on which the novel rests will collapse. And if I can't write the novel, then why am I here?

While I'm in my meeting, Sadie sends me a FaceTime request, which I ignore. Leaving, though, I see that I have a dozen messages from her, including a screenshot of a statement released on one of her social media accounts, which I stop on the sidewalk to read. In it, Sadie commands her many followers to stop engaging with any work by the famous white feminist director Jill and I were talking about earlier, the one who recently publicly defended the white TV writer accused of raping the Black actress. Sadie also writes that she decided to publish this callout after reading the young actress's account of her rape at the hands of the TV writer "due to its similarity to something that happened to a friend of hers when we were both in school."

I've been staying in Brooklyn with my old friend Charlotte, and on the train to her apartment, I read the rest of the statement, which Sadie has also posted to Facebook. Styled like a press release and detailing a number of complaints against the controversial director, one part reads, "A close friend was raped by a powerful, white man we both knew when we were in college. . . . It was never really talked about and this man continues to maintain a very high status within the creative community. Who knows who else he has done this to? I will always regret not speaking out about it at the time and wonder if I could have done more to help my friend process what happened."

The friend Sadie is talking about, I understand after a moment, is me. She's referencing what happened in college in that Upper East Side apartment, where our mutual acquaintance shoved his penis into my body while I slept. Sadie is comparing what that person did to me to what was done to the young actress, drawing a connection between the boy and the famous feminist director. But what I can't understand is why. In the days after, Sadie was very much there for me, and she has nothing to feel bad about. I certainly don't feel bad about it anymore—I never think about it.

That evening, I'm on my way to spend Thanksgiving with Ethan's family, and I only barely have time to grab my things from Charlotte's before I have to catch the bus. On the ride to Boston, I open my laptop and edit a scene in *The Anatomy Book* in which Mark tries to talk to Laura about the discovery of dark energy, then close it again, queasy with uncertainty about how any of this could ever possibly matter.

ETHAN PICKS ME UP AT South Station with the dog in the passenger seat. We drive to his parents' house in the suburbs. Over dinner, Vivian, Ethan's four-year-old niece, tells us about her best friend, Madeleine, who touched the water in the toilet tank at school. Ethan's mom offers to take me wedding dress shopping. Ethan's dad watches a Western on the couch with Ethan's brother and sister. Like I do every year, I surrender to their goodwill, falling asleep on the couch with their cockapoo draped over my lap.

I wake up on Thanksgiving Day, light streaming in through Ethan's childhood bedroom window. We take the dog down to the forest behind his parents' house. She streaks across a frozen meadow, happy to be off-leash. Chasing her, we come face-to-face with a wolf-sized dog with a battered bell hanging around its neck. All three of us freeze in fear, certain Larry Bird will be eaten. But the bigger dog only shakes its bell and takes off toward an owner hidden somewhere in the woods.

When we get back to Ethan's parents' house, I find out Sadie's statement against the director has migrated off Facebook and onto the home pages of mainstream news outlets. Sadie is popular online, and several journalists follow her. In the odd, slow days around the holiday, her public statement makes headlines. Stories citing Sadie's accusations appear on the BBC.com, in the *Guardian*, in *People*, in *New York* magazine, *Variety*, the *Hollywood Reporter*, and the *Daily Beast*. Celebrity authors and then actual celebrities signal-boost her message. People I know text me links to articles quoting Sadie asking if I'm seeing her name everywhere the way they are, asking what I think. Sadie calls me multiple times and I send each call to voicemail.

The rage Sadie's statement inspires online is seductive and powerful. It fuels itself and sparks think pieces in smaller publications that go viral on Twitter and serve to fuel it further. The filmmaker at the center of the maelstrom, who found great success very young and, some believe, undeservedly, posts a written apology and retreats from the public eye. I read the comments under each article and feel my heart beat faster. This is the closest I'll ever be—or ever want to be—to the zeitgeist. Sadie's literary influence is now so great she accidentally sparked a brief, but powerful, national conversation about something that happened to me.

All during this time, Sadie sends me mortified messages that I read without answering. I don't know why. It's just that, if Sadie hadn't alerted me to the post, the truth is, I would never have known I was the one she was talking about. This is because I don't remember ever really thinking of what happened as rape. On any other night, I might have slept with that boy willingly, and he must have known that. And besides, as soon as I told him to stop, he stopped. Becoming part of a larger conversation about sexual assault doesn't feel like the kind of thing I should get to have conflicting feelings about, but I am conflicted, a little. For Sadie and for the people involved, this boy is only one small part of a much larger story, and maybe what happened to me deserves to be its own story, or maybe I don't want it to be a story at all. Nobody asked me, and it seems as if someone should have. I don't want people on the internet to decide to what degree my own experience determines how I feel.

I try to funnel my anxiety into my manuscript, attempt to look at it critically, from a distance. The scene I'm revising hinges on Laura's all-consuming wish to find Mark. She's unaware Mark is searching for a different Laura in a different universe who is also searching for him. But any interest I ever had in fixing Mark is gone. This book is meant to be a book about urgent desire, but I'm repulsed by Mark, which is why the novel won't work.

Rereading the first chapter for the thousandth time, a memory jogs loose in my brain. I know what's been bothering me about the character. It's his name. Mark is also the name of the boy in the Upper East Side apartment, the boy Sadie is talking about now in her statement. And it isn't as if I'd forgotten Mark's name. It's only that I never thought about Mark at all. Now, it appears he took up residence in my subconscious only to burst forth as the main character in a novel I can't finish and that is slowly driving me to despair. I never understood why I hated the character of Mark so much, but could also not excise him from the story. Now I do. The immediate result of this revelation is that whatever power I'd gained over Mark and what he did by never thinking about him is ripped violently away. My agency was taken from me then, and it is being taken from me now. An anger born in 2007 wells violently up in the present. I want all of my rage to be directed at Mark, and I'm confused by how much of it feels aimed at Sadie.

...

"TAKE IT LIKE A WOMAN," my mother would say, if I tried to tell her about what was happening right now. And then, as if by thinking of her I have conjured her, she calls me and—my mistake—I answer the phone. She is in the middle of a sentence, and I put her on speaker and listen.

"I don't know if you understand, but Lance is ruthless. He's criminally harassing me and I went to the police and I hope they started a case and he burns my vagina and right now I have a cut that almost goes down to my chin because he lasers my lip or he lasers my vagina or he lasers my head. I can't lie comfortably or sit comfortably at all and that really scares me, and I can't see how he would be so vicious or vindictive as to include you in this effort to harass me. I don't put anything past him. I don't want to bring you into something you shouldn't be involved in, but I was so worried when I woke up and I texted you and I wanted to let you know—"

I set the phone on the floor and sit down on Ethan's childhood bed a few feet away from it, but still I can hear her. "You were a young girl in a dream I had and I was sitting in the back seat of the car, and I could feel your head going through the car door window and I saw glass everywhere and as you hit the window I woke up and I was, I couldn't breathe, I felt so nervous, I started praying, trying to figure out what exactly—"

Ethan's mother is calling my name from downstairs. We have an appointment to go look at wedding dresses. "Okay, Mom, I'm sorry, I know, it sounds so painful, I'll call you," I tell her. "I have to go."

The air outside is cold and wet. We drive past tall pines onto the highway and on to an upscale mall in Newton. The saleswoman has blond streaks in her brown hair and a very round face. "We're not like traditional wedding stores. We're very different," she says. The dresses she brings me have names: Octavia, Freesia, Kyla. I try on a dress that looks like a cake, so stiff and heavy it stands up on its own. I stare at myself in the dress and decide I will stop thinking. I will not consider. I will not remember. I will not re-hash. I am amazed by how well this works, and I wish a therapist, a relative, Ethan, anyone, had told me how beneficial it could be to simply stop the perpetual whirr of the brain, though at the same time, I can see how, once introduced to the concept, one might be tempted to stop it for good.

ETHAN HAS AN INVITATION TO the Tallinn Black Nights Film Festival in Estonia, where an independent film he produced is premiering. He arranges for me to get a festival pass as well. We fly into a city like something out of Kafka's short stories—the pointed roofs of the houses all leaning at improbable angles over wet streets. We watch movies in rooms carved out of medieval stone. One film is about characters in a small town stuck in a time loop, and I find myself enthralled. The director's name is Alex, and he is coolly attractive in a way that would have intimidated me if I'd met him under other circumstances.

"How are you still single?" I ask him at the closing night party, which is held in a freezing Soviet-era warehouse the size of an airplane hangar. "You should let me fix you up with one of our friends."

I've been drinking and I'm talking too loud. Over Alex's shoulder, I see Ethan's ears perk up. He senses something off.

"You think he's cute, don't you?" he whispers, joining us. "You're flirting."

Before I can answer, two other directors we've befriended appear and sweep Ethan off to take pictures in the photo booth. I continue talking to Alex.

"I was in a serious relationship a few years ago. But it ended," he tells me.

"Why?"

"Well, it was complicated. My mother killed herself—"

I feel myself go cold all over. "What?"

"It made dating difficult."

"What happened?" I ask again.

"She'd been sick for about a decade. We tried to get her help. She was in and out of hospitals, but she didn't believe us that anything was wrong, and you can't forcibly commit an adult—"

"Unless she's a danger to herself," I say. "I know."

"And we didn't know how much danger she was in until it was too late, I guess."

"I'm so sorry," I say, realizing I haven't said this yet. Then I start to cry. I tell him about my mother.

"Just try to enjoy being with her when she'll let you, and when you can," he says. He gives me a hug. He's warm and skinnier than I expected. I can feel his rib cage through his jacket. The fact of this other body against mine surprises me so much I shrink back, not used to such close contact with anyone other than Ethan. I see, over Alex's shoulder, Ethan staring.

We leave the party and walk to the hotel to get our bags and head to the airport for our early morning flight. Ethan is clearly annoyed. Alex is the only person I spoke to at the party all night.

"What?" I say.

Ethan names a beautiful novelist acquaintance of mine. Her photos in magazines are all marked by a soft, sweet, white feminine vulnerability that makes me want to squeeze her head until it pops. "What if I spent all night talking to her at a party for something you'd written?" he asks.

"He lost his mother," I say. "She killed herself. I've never met anyone who went through that before. At least not who would talk about it."

Mollified, Ethan is quiet. A few minutes later, he speaks again to point out the part of the city where an abandoned chemical plant served as the primary filming location for *Stalker*. The ground was still poisoned with chemical runoff. Within a decade much of the cast and crew would develop terminal cancer, including Tarkovsky himself.

We finish the ride in respectful silence, but once we get to the airport, Ethan says, "Also, by the way, don't you think it's a little too cold out for such a short dress? I don't know why you would even bring that here."

"You absolutely do not ever get to tell me what to wear." I nearly spit the words. "And I know we have plans to go to your family's house for Christmas, but I'm not going. I have a family too."

We're fighting past each other about two different things that, awkwardly, neither one of us wants to articulate. He thinks I have a crush on Alex, and I don't. I want to visit my mother for Christmas and think he's against this, but he's not. Or I want to want this, feel guilty for not wanting it enough to have fought for it before, want to enjoy being with my mother while I can, even though I don't enjoy being with her at all. I would much prefer to be in Ethan's big house in the woods with his parents and siblings and nieces and nephews and their seemingly boundless supply of love.

ELEVEN

SADIE CALLS AS SOON AS I get back to L.A. I look at her name on my caller ID and send the call to voicemail as I have ten times before. She leaves a message. "Hey, I can't come by on Saturday night," she says like we're in the middle of a conversation which we are not. I have not suggested any night for her to come by at all. "But I could do Friday. Let me know."

I know what she's doing. Cutting through the bullshit. Forcing her way in. Refusing to allow me to close her out. Part of me is grateful for her stubbornness. It isn't as if she used my name in her public statement. Her intention was good. She wasn't trying to hurt me. She hasn't hurt me. I'm not hurt, exactly. I don't know what I am. I only know some small, dramatic part of me feels as if she's inadvertently committed a moral transgression so vast as to be incomprehensible. I text her back. Sure, I say, Friday is good.

As soon as Sadie enters my apartment she dissolves into tears. "I'm sorry," she says. "I had an emotional freak-out. I shouldn't have used what happened to you like that. It wasn't okay. You've been a good friend to me, but if you don't want to be my friend anymore, I understand." She looks tired and pretty, her eyes red around the edges and her nose puffy. I walk into the kitchen, open the cabinet, pull out rice cakes and almond butter.

"You hungry?" I ask. I spread the almond butter out with a spoon, and it feels good to be able to do this one thing, to take care of her in this way. But back in the living room, Sadie feeds almond butter to the dog, and some of it gets on the couch, which I will now have to clean, and I seethe.

I make small talk to get her out of my apartment, to put this moment out of its misery. I tell her about editing *The Anatomy Book*, about how paralyzed I feel about its flaws and how much I want to be working on a different book, more in line with the oratorio, about my mother and everything that has happened to her this past year.

"Then write that," Sadie says.

"I feel like I can't abandon *The Anatomy Book* until it's finished or at least goes out on submission," I say. "It's like a tumor, a parasite sucking all the nutrients out of me, but if I try to cut it out, I'll die."

"You say that a lot," she says. "And you've been saying it for years. You have to think about your career. Like, what kind of writer do you want to be? Who's your model?"

"I don't know." The question sounds absurd. "What kind of writer do you want to be?"

"Toni Morrison," she says, immediately, and once again I find myself in thrall to her absolute inability to even pretend at a lack of confidence.

"Victor LaValle," I say, trying to imitate her quickness. "Helen Oyeyemi."

"Why don't you send me your novel and I'll send it to my agent,"

Sadie says. "If she doesn't like it, no harm, no foul, and if she does, well . . . you have a new option."

"I'll think about it." Sadie's agent is an important name in publishing, and if I accept and something comes of it, she'll have done me yet another life-changing favor. Everything will go back to the way it always was, with her two steps ahead, tossing a hand behind her so I can almost keep up.

"My story . . . what happened . . . wasn't yours," I say. I feel the words pulse out of me, propulsive and angry as a fist. But they land softly, if they land at all. Sadie looks at me, a little amused, and I feel stupid and melodramatic, hate how false trying to express myself authentically feels. "You don't get to use what happened to me for yourself. For your own anger. I worked hard to get where I am, and it isn't fair for that to be negated. For me to be made into a victim in a story when that's not what I am."

"I know," Sadie says. "I know where you come from."

But she doesn't. She's never been to the house in Riverside Terrace. She doesn't know what the air felt like in summer or how heavy the sky was just before it rained. She doesn't know about my fear that my life will curl in on itself and I will end up back there with my mother, the two of us enveloped in silence. I want to tell her about all of it, not in those words, but in better ones. At the same time, I wonder how much she wishes I understood about her. What parts of her am I blind to, too hurt to be curious about?

ETHAN AND I GO TO dinner at the Line hotel in Koreatown. Things still feel strange between us, not least because we've not fully addressed the fight in Estonia that made them strange in the first place. That night, I'm meeting an old friend of his for the first time, a costume designer named Filipa and her husband, who are visiting from Canada for work. Filipa and I like each other right away, fall into easy conversation about Black hair products. She tells me about her daylong flat-ironing process, and I commiserate, tell her I could never straighten my own hair because it's fine and gets tangled easily and I'm too impatient not to tear out the knots.

"You know, some of my friends think Sarah is mixed," Ethan says. He's trying to join our conversation, referring to the medium brown color of my skin, but the remark appears to come from nowhere.

"That's slavery for you!" says Filipa after a quiet moment. I cringe a little, internally, and pour myself a second glass of wine.

Ethan goes to the bathroom. I count slowly in my head to ten. My breathing returns to normal. A few minutes later, he comes back. He points to his head. "Why didn't anyone tell me I have an Afro?" His hair has expanded into a curly halo around his face in the humidity.

Not in front of my new Black friend! I want to shout at him, as if it's my fault he would say something so stupid. I know he's not trying to upset anyone, but in this specific situation, I feel as if I'm in charge of educating him and I have failed. Filipa looks over at me briefly and laughs a little. Is it my imagination or do I hear pity in the sound?

I know I could drop it here and the night would be fine—these are Ethan's friends, after all, not mine, they've known him longer, and no one seems to be bothered but me—but as the food arrives and conversation moves on, I find myself spinning into a rage I can't quell.

"Is there a reason you're being so embarrassing?" I ask Ethan.

"I'm always embarrassing," he says with a smile.

It's true he is often embarrassing, and besides, it's not as if I haven't embarrassed him in public multiple times. I remember a dinner party at which, nervous, I drank too much champagne and picked a fight with a famous screenwriter about whether Julie Delpy had written and directed the film *Before Sunrise*. I would not back down even when presented with compelling evidence that I was wrong. Still, half of me wants to flip the table, and the other half is exerting all its energy to stop me.

"YOU CAN'T BE LIKE THIS forever," Ethan says when we get home. I'm trying to avoid speaking to him, and I won't tell him why, because I don't know what I'll do or say. I push past him into the hallway, go into and out of the bathroom and then to the bedroom. There are only so many doors in our tiny apartment, but I will slam them all.

"Aren't you," Ethan says, following me from room to room, "on some level, much too old to be acting like this? Talk to me."

There's so much about who I am and what is happening to me now—with my mother, with my grandmother, with Sadie—that Ethan doesn't know and that I can't be bothered to explain.

"I'm angry because you don't care about me. You don't love me. You don't support me."

Ethan looks frustrated. I watch him consider refuting each

accusation point by point, and then deciding not to. "Where is this coming from?" he asks.

I trip a little bit coming out of the bathroom for the second time. I had two cocktails at dinner, and the four of us split a bottle of wine. I need Ethan to stop talking to me, I need him to stop trying to figure out what's wrong by talking it out and fixing it. But he's incapable of letting a conflict go unresolved. So my only option is to repeat all the words my mother is always saying to me in my head.

I tell him he's spoiled, that he's never had any real problems, that he has no idea what it means to feel pain, that he's selfish and thoughtless and careless. I recognize the look on his face as a look I used to give my own mother and the feeling is as if, in stabbing someone else, I've felt the blade drive itself into my own heart. An image of my mother's face, contorted in anger, her hand raised to strike, fingernails curved into actual claws, flashes in my mind. But even that is not enough to make me stop.

"In the morning, when you're sober, you're going to apologize and I'm going to forgive you, but I need you to know that what you're saying hurts," Ethan says.

I already feel terrible, but the feeling is no match for my fury. I put on the running shoes he gave me for Christmas and jog drunkenly outside into the darkness. I don't know how to fix this. I feel incredibly alone.

Sadie would understand. She's known me the longest. Knows how to listen and be sympathetic without telling me what I want to hear. But I haven't really forgiven her yet. If I text her now, our relationship will regress to the mean—out of fear of losing her, I'll be lulled back into complacency.

I think about a time before I met Ethan, when I used to wander around Hollywood in a dress I bought from Goodwill for two dollars. I made friends that way, drifting into parties off the sidewalk or into bars, anywhere I heard laughter and music. Once, a boy I'd hooked up with after a dinner party spotted me on Fairfax Avenue, picked me up, and took me with him to Las Vegas with his friends. He disappeared once we got to the tables, and I spent the weekend with the couple we'd driven up with listening to comedy specials and shrooming. I came home pleased with the new friends I'd made, unharmed, feeling protected. On my walks back then in Los Angeles, psychics were constantly pulling me aside to tell me I had a deep energy, that I should come see them for a reading. I knew better than to believe them—I was young, female, alone, and they assumed I was an easy target—but it made me feel special, and I let it. There is a part of me still out there, going home with strangers and staying up late, skinny and haunting the area around Fountain and Santa Monica. I could protect Ethan from myself by finding that girl who had no attachments to anyone and trying to become her again.

I DO A READING AT a bar in Frogtown for a literary journal of the essay I wrote about the white supremacist in Houston. After I read, the journal's editor, Phillip, and I share a drink. He mentions his girlfriend, Emma, the translator I met at Sadie's Airbnb. She's having the same kind of stomach pain I used to get. I cured mine during a residency at Yaddo, three weeks during which I was supposed to be writing that I spent, instead, researching cures for IBS. I tell him I have suggestions—peppermint oil capsules for pain and a natural antibiotic—and give him my number so Emma can call me. He thanks me and, feeling more accomplished than I have in weeks, I tell him he and Emma should come over for dinner soon.

That weekend, Ethan's brother and his wife come to visit Los Angeles with their six-month-old daughter. James is a taller, more relaxed version of Ethan, and Katarina is sophisticated and straightforward. We take them to dinner at a café down the street and share a basket of waffle fries on the patio.

If you're angry with me, Sadie texts me, I think you owe me an explanation.

The text comes out of nowhere. Our last few exchanges have been cordial and meaningless, a quick back-and-forth about a celebrity-branded leave-in conditioner. I place my phone face down on the table. But I can't help looking at it again a few minutes later. Two more messages have come through. Both radiate anger.

She recently saw Phillip and found out I invited him and Emma over for dinner, which she didn't appreciate. Why am I spending time with her friends when I am constantly dodging Sadie herself?

And it's true. Although I've messaged with Sadie, I've ignored any overtures at making in-person plans. She knows I'm avoiding her and she's mad about it and I don't know how to navigate this situation. I only know how to be unfailingly polite, to quietly hope whatever bad thing is happening will eventually stop. I type out a vague apology, then delete it without sending it and turn my phone off for the night. I ignore Sadie because I don't want to confront whatever it is that's actually wrong. From my experience with my mother, it appears I have learned nothing.

...

150

ON SUNDAY, ETHAN AND I go with James and Katarina and their baby to celebrate Easter at a friend's house in Burbank. As soon as we arrive, Sadie texts me again.

Um, hi? she writes. There's a threat in the words that makes me feel deranged.

At an Easter egg hunt right now. I can talk soon. I hit send and put my phone in my purse, afraid of how she'll respond. We are at one of those L.A. parties for creative children put together expertly by artists who build film sets for a living, who belong to Hollywood unions. The moment is strange and idyllic, and under other circumstances, I would send Sadie a picture of the elaborate pastel streamers and the giant papier-mâché bunnies and she would draft the perfect half-mocking, half-admiring response. In another time of our friendship, she might even have shown up, invited by me, and left, hours later, beloved by everyone.

Can we talk? Are you around? Probably best not to prolong this process, she writes.

Ethan wants to know why I'm not looking for eggs. I text Sadie to back off and tell her I'll call her in a little while. She tells me I've made my feelings on the matter clear and that I should not bother.

IN THE MORNING, WORKING ON the oratorio's third movement, I look through a list of all the places the Jet Propulsion Laboratory has helped send satellites and rockets to forge a path for humans. I make the list into a song, starting with the closest satellite and ending with a list of the names of the deserts on Mars. I imagine Reese's music going up and up through the roof of Disney Hall

151

into the night, into the mountains that surround the city, rising forever into the sky.

An email from Sadie pops up in my inbox. The first I've heard from her since yesterday.

I told you before how I remembered it. This entire book is a chronicle of how I remember it. Now Sadie wants to tell me what she remembers. Her version of recent events is, as is to be expected, very different from mine.

She writes that she's been reflecting on our relationship in the time since I refused to take her calls after her public statement, and she's come to the conclusion that I've slipped into a world of Los Angeles writers that she isn't—and doesn't want to be—a part of. She finds my disappearance into the literary world here, which she calls vapid and unserious, painful, because she's always thought of me as a serious person. To be blunt, she writes, I thought you were better than that. She's frustrated at the fact that I've chosen to associate with and take advice from writers she believes she's better than. If you want to write real literature, you're not going to do it surrounded by these people.

She was never actually upset because of my wanting to spend time with Emma and Phillip, but because of how many times she feels I've failed to stick up for her, given how much she's done for me. My choosing to reach out to Emma and not her is only the most recent example, and to be honest, she's beginning to feel used by me. She's felt that way more and more as her profile has risen along with her book's success, and it hurts even worse when the source of the feeling is a friend. She also believes I've been taking digs at her—digs I might not even realize I'm making. Part of the reason she sent so many urgent texts, the tone of which she apologizes for, was because she wanted to make me aware.

When you were here with Emma, I started talking about politics, and you snapped at me out of nowhere, "You're being defensive!" I don't need to mention that the incident with Kate was also about politics, and your response to that was to also scream at me, "She wasn't being racist!" when she insulted me first.

As politics have become a more significant part of her life, it's become more and more difficult for her to spend time with me. She finds my attitude about Bernie Sanders demeaning and condescending, not to mention screwed up, since I'm in the majority, while she's threatened and put at risk for advocating for her beliefs. She also believes my positioning places me "squarely on the wrong side of history."

At this point, I don't feel I deserve to be ignored in this way. I can't count how many times I've dropped everything at the suggestion that something was going wrong for you. I honestly can't imagine receiving a text like the one I sent you and not at least trying to figure out what was wrong.

She'll be traveling abroad soon and believes this break will naturally lead to the end of our friendship. If I genuinely want to talk, she's open to it, but she won't be reaching out to me anymore and requests that I no longer reach out to her for favors or advice.

I would appreciate if you . . . tread lightly when it comes to our common friendships, especially the ones that I have made available to you. I will not speak badly about you personally, and I will never stand in your way professionally. But I absolutely cannot help you anymore.

She knows I have a lot of great things coming up in my life and she's sad she won't be a part of them, but our friendship is hurting her and I've left her no choice but to end it.

I read the email again. Each sentence feels like a physical assault. She wants me to argue, wants me to tell her why I'm angry, to make her apologize again and again. The fact that I prefer to pretend nothing happened makes her feel like I don't care. And still, I can't do the one thing that might fix it, which is pick up the phone and talk to her. I'm too afraid she'll yell at me, or, worse, that she won't pick up at all. That she'll see my name on the caller ID and ignore it, the way my mother used to.

In another world, I call, she answers, we have the fight. But in this one, I write back to Sadie to say that I respect her decision and wish her all the best.

TWELVE

ETHAN AND I HAVE PLANS to visit a potential wedding venue in Paso Robles, a ranch owned by his friends Ted and Diana. We will swim in their pool and play with their dogs and have dinner overlooking their vineyard. I eat a dark chocolate–covered coffee bean infused with THC before we leave Los Angeles, and by the time we arrive, the day is wobbling all around me. The liver in their German shorthaired pointer's bowl looks alive, as if the pieces of it are crawling over one another. A dead velvet-furred mole I find in a garden near the entrance to the property seems to have been planted there as a sign. The red ants everywhere appear to be carrying messages, and even Diana seems to be speaking in code.

"I love watching the sun set over these eucalyptus trees," she says. I stare at her beautiful features but can't make them into a face. Larry Bird pads over to nose my hand, looking for a treat and stretches out flat by the pool. I've been watching her tame the pointer, who is twice her size. Now she bares her teeth and growls because he has come too close. She wanders off into the cool darkness of the house.

"Humans to dogs are just hairless monkeys," I accidentally say out loud.

"We're more than that," Diana says, sounding alarmed.

"What do you think a dog would do if it saw a hairless monkey?" asks Ethan, who is drinking a beer in a lawn chair. A seedpod explodes with a sound like a gunshot. The seeds scatter across the warm patio tile. Diana gazes moodily over the pool. I'm bumming her out. She doesn't know what to do with me.

"You two set a date yet?" she says.

I hear a commotion coming from inside and race back across the yard, too stoned to move quickly, feeling as if I'm pushing back against a wall of water. Larry Bird has gotten into a fight with the pointer over a knuckle bone. The other dog bit her ear, and it's bleeding. By the time I get there, Ethan has separated them. Diana helps me clean the wound and I lie with Larry Bird against my chest in the guest room, feeling her small body tremble, Ethan beside us. The bleeding stops as quickly as it started. She falls asleep, but I'm still crying. Holding her, I repeat for Ethan all the things Sadie wrote, taking pleasure in knowing the email by heart. What I want—what I think I want—I tell him, is for everyone who has ever hurt me to fall in line and explain to me explicitly what I did to deserve it. But they aren't here. The only person here is Ethan, and he is growing tired.

"What Sadie did is not about you. It's about her. She's probably feeling vulnerable. It's psychologically dangerous to go from being normal to famous so fast. And she's taking it out on you. She might not even know it. You always think other people know so much more than you. But they don't. People grow, and sometimes in the process, they fuck up. You're the collateral damage here."

"No," I say, "I mean it. I want you to tell me what's wrong with me. Be honest. Say it straight to my face."

"Well." His brow furrows. "Nobody ever knows what you're thinking, because you won't say. People assume you're quietly judging them. No one likes that. You feel sorry for yourself a lot. You don't always consider other people's feelings. And, I mean, when was the last time you apologized to anyone? You always expect people to give you a pass, but you're so quick to cut people out when they piss you off. You think all these crazy things are wrong with you, but you won't look your actual faults in the face." He pauses. "You're self-involved. You're not very interested in other people except in ways that directly pertain to you or your writing."

"Sure," I say softly. All of this sounds right. It is exactly who I am. But none of it is anything I plan to change.

"You never stick around to have the fight. There's something in your ego that won't allow you to hear what you don't want to. You disappear inside your own head."

I nod and stare out the window into Ted and Diana's vast yard. "What if we said fuck it and ran away somewhere?" I say. "What if we bought a house out here?"

"That's exactly what I'm talking about." Ethan says. "We can't afford a house. What would that even fix?"

"I don't know," I say. But I do. I am trying to get away from Ethan's words, from my book, from my agent, from Sadie, from my belief that I drove my mother mad and that I drove Sadie away and that I will do the same thing to Ethan. From the depression I'm always trying to give the slip.

But then I remember the way my mother always told me how much she wanted to run away to Atlanta, where she would start a business. Newark, where she would be a flight attendant. Berkeley, where I would go to college. West Africa, where she would find out which country she's really from. We were always going to go somewhere, and it was always going to fix all her problems. But we never left, and nothing ever got fixed. How did I fall so smoothly into the channels carved out for me?

All I've done is resist.

The resistance led me here.

"Are you spacing out again?" Ethan says. "You'd do anything to avoid reality. Work on your novel. Finish it. Move on. You can do it. I believe in you."

I GO BACK TO SUPPORT group, where we learn about the LEAP system for breaking through to mentally ill loved ones: Listen, Empathize, Ask Questions, and Partner. The instructor calls on volunteers to discuss our weeks. I raise my hand. I'm here to talk about Sadie, not my mother. If I listen to Sadie and empathize with her, I think, she will answer my questions and then we will be partners. I will access the full extent of my humanity and I will use it to force her to access hers.

The others watch me, blank-faced, as I recite the email out loud for them. These people have real problems. Relatives suffering from pervasive, incurable delusions, loved ones they can't save. Mothers and fathers and brothers and sisters they take care of because everyone else in the family has given up. I know they don't care about my stupid fight with my stupid friend. But I tell them anyway, about the text messages, about the fact that I never picked up and she kept calling. I don't mention that I did the same thing to my mother, ignoring her calls and texts for over a year, before she lost her mind.

"Tell her you're sorry she feels that way," says a woman who shared a story about a sister who calls to accuse her of imagined crimes dozens of times a day. The woman thinks what I want is a way to end the conversation, to get away from Sadie, the way this woman wants to get away from her sister. But what I want is for someone to tell me what I keep doing that pushes everyone I care for away so that I can stop doing it. Barring that, what I want is to be somebody else.

THE ORATORIO IS ABOUT TO premiere. I go with the composer to a studio in Pasadena to record interviews for NPR affiliates in Houston and L.A. and do an interview with the *Los Angeles Times*. I force myself to sound smarter than I believe I am, but hear myself like the striving student I've always been, saying all the right things to get an A-plus, to make the teacher like me because I make her job easy. I talk about the cyclical nature of human history, about how storytelling is the opposite of division, how art opens up the spectator and lets itself in, which is a line I stole from an author I heard on a podcast.

The reporters appear mostly unimpressed. I get the sense I am disappointing them. That what they want from me is abrasiveness, friction, good quotes, something that might cause a stir. That the expectation is that I will be more emotional, not academic. Everything Reese says sounds this way, honest and open and deeply *felt*, and I wonder why everything I say comes out caked in a layer of mud that renders it senseless. I wonder how Sadie would do each interview if she were here instead of me. Sadie, with her confident regality. Instead of me, with my polite, high-pitched voice that always makes me sound as if I am asking the question instead of answering it.

On the day of the concert, I panic about what to wear. None of my clothes seem right. I decide to go shopping. I go to a department store and buy the first dress I try on, which is long and white and matronly. Next, I get my hair blown out but can't pull up the picture on the salon's Wi-Fi of the celebrity I want to look like—Naomie Harris—so end up with middle-aged church lady curls, like James Brown. I step outside into a day so humid it's immediately as if I never did anything to my hair at all.

Only when I try on the dress at my apartment do I understand it was designed for a woman much older than me. It's an ugly gown with a collar that chokes me at the base of my neck. I turn this way and that in the mirror. No matter what I do, I look like I've aged twenty years. But it's too late to fix it now. I hurry downtown to the concert hall.

I'm excited because a classical-radio DJ whose program I used to listen to every morning on my way to work is going to interview me and the composer at a pre-concert panel. But for most of the panel, I sit in silence, head swiveling back and forth, while he addresses questions to the composer and our researcher, ignoring me. It dawns on me that he's forgotten my name and so can't address me directly, and I interject then to say the soundbites I've memo-rized but that I'm not sure I believe in. "This piece represents such hope."

Still, the performance, after everything, is staggering. I feel the energy in the room, the way it concentrates and spreads, the au-dience breathing as one, all of us nodes in a network. The music moves through each of us like an impulse through synapses in a brain. In the third movement, I've included quotes from the tech-nologists we interviewed in Los Angeles.

> *Mars is cold, but we can warm it.*
> *We can compress the atmosphere.*
> *We can harvest the moon.*
> *And then on Mars*
> *we'll finally have something that resembles a home.*
> *Where do we go beyond Earth?*
> *Gale Crater, Gusev Crater, Elysium Planitia,*
> *Alba Mons, Olympus Mons, Hellas Planitia.*

A soloist accidentally skips my favorite line (*I have a friend / who wants to die in space / you'll see Earth as you're going*). It's hard to tell if the rest of the words are landing the way I mean for them to. But before the singing ends, I hear someone near me whisper, "Oh my God," and someone else lets out an audible gasp, and that is when I know we've done it. The audience rises to its feet. I climb down to the stage in my ugly dress. I can feel myself shake as we bow.

I go back to Reese's dressing room and lie down on the floor. Reese lies next to me. She keeps calling the audience "generous."

She wonders whether the standing ovation was real. She watched from the sound booth so couldn't experience what it sounded like for the audience. I tell her what happened to the crowd, how all of us breathed in together. I tell her I'd been worried the text was ponderous but that onstage it worked. We eat pizza and take shots of whiskey. And at the after-party in the donors' lounge, I embarrass myself in front of a wealthy couple who helped fund the performance by being self-deprecating to the point of nihilism. They ask me questions and I hear myself answer too quickly, too chirpily, not sure what to do when confronted by their concerned stares. Who is this girl? I imagine them wondering. Where did she come from? And I want to wave my hands in front of them and shout: Look! In spite of everything, I'm here.

The morning after the show there is nothing in me but happiness, like a thousand doors thrown open. I sit in a coffee shop in West Hollywood and work on *The Anatomy Book*, feeling capable of so much more. Sadie's email fades. The success of last night feels like a step away from my mother's destiny, a step toward the creation of my own.

THE REVIEW THAT COMES OUT in the *Los Angeles Times*, however, is not positive. I read it at Ethan's desk, set up in the cramped corner of the living room. The critic compliments the music but did not like my libretto. "It is possible—as John Adams and Peter Sellars have shown, and Julia Wolfe in her oratorio, 'Anthracite Fields'—to create profound musical expression around documentary material. Some of the libretto's historical lines, especially from Memphis, really do sing, but too often there is conventional wisdom. When we get to [the third movement about our trajectory from Los Angeles to Mars and beyond], it's basically TED talk."[33]

"TED talk?" I say.

Ethan makes a face. "It's only a bad review," he says.

"I'm really sad," I say to Ethan, and the words sound stale in my mouth. The pain washing over me isn't unlike the pain I felt when I read Sadie's email. I've gotten what I deserved for trying to rise above my station. I am back where I belong. Supposed to lose and losing.

"How can anyone tell if classical music is good or not?" Ethan asks. "How does anyone even know? We don't know anything about opera."

"It's because he's white," I say. "It's because he's a white man! That critic doesn't want me to be in the club. No one wants me to be in their club."

"You're not being very nice to yourself," Ethan observes, then yawns and the dog yawns too, which makes Ethan laugh. "Would you stop?" he continues. "It's like you went on a cooking show and you're mad you didn't win even though you barely ever cook and you don't even know if you're good at it because you're not, like, a food critic either." Lost in his metaphor, he gives up. "Also fuck that guy. He critiques opera for a living. Of course he's bitter. He's irrelevant."

Ethan goes to the hall closet where he keeps press clippings from his films. He comes back with the print edition of the *New York Times* from the week his first feature came out. In it, the critic argues his characters don't seem to come from anywhere, suggesting the filmmaker knows nothing about coming-of-age in a small town. The entire film was shot in the small town outside Boston where Ethan spent his adolescence. But he isn't bothered.

"You know what most people are going to remember about this?" Ethan crows. "*Not* that I got a bad review. But that a still photo from my film is in color in the *New York* fucking *Times*."

The review of my oratorio includes a line suggesting I grew up in Houston during the oil boom and bust of the seventies. I was born in 1985. It's the cursed dress, my sausage curls that made me look like a mother of the bride. Ethan gets fed up with my nonsense and goes to bed, but I stay awake and read the review repeatedly, driving it into my brain like a spike.

The next morning, when I go back to the *Los Angeles Times* website, I discover Ethan has written a long, mean comment under the review—I know it was him, because the fake name he used was "Larry Bird"—offering a point-by-point rebuttal of everything the critic said, and I force him to delete it before anyone sees.

IN SUPPORT GROUP, WE DO an exercise meant to simulate the voices people with schizophrenia hear in their heads. The point is to prove aural hallucinations are real. Our loved ones hear voices we can't hear, feel certain they have access to a reality we don't, and that is why they look, to us, as if they cannot function. The exercise, which involves a partner who shouts voices into my ear while I try to follow instructions for completion of a simple task, is meant to replicate their auditory delusions. Mona, the woman assigned to be my partner, is witchy, with huge blue eyes, and is a little too good at this. As she hollers the scripted lines (*they hate you, they want you to die*) and I try to complete the task (drawing a many-sided figure on a sheet of graph paper), I start to cry. Mona laughs awkwardly. The exercise makes us all feel bad.

"Given this," says the support group leader, "how should we communicate with our loved ones?" We spend the rest of the class practicing starting sentences with "I feel" and "I wish" and "I would like."

JILL WRITES TO ASK FOR the new draft of my book. I send it. The following day, she writes back saying she'll finish it immediately and wants to put it out on submission as soon as possible. We set a time for a call, but she doesn't keep the appointment, so I email her again. This time I don't receive an answer.

I PARTICIPATE IN A READING at an art gallery displaying paintings of a gay Adolf Hitler joyfully penetrated by many pale pink cocks. After I read, a poet in an overpriced designer peasant dress reads a series of very bad poems. *Why am I doing this?* I wonder, listening to the girl read her awful poetry in her awful poet voice. Writers on those websites that publish essays purporting to teach other people how to become writers are always asking what fiction can do in the current political moment, and I think now the answer is nothing. Following the literary world feels more and more like watching the fragile children of aristocrats gingerly explore their talents while their friends applaud and the world around them burns. I feel like all of what most writers say is bullshit and all readers know this and are quietly indulging them. Some get indulged more than others, and everyone else fights to bask in their stupid glory.

How much more of my life can I throw away? Writing, I feel like an addict most of the time, chasing the pleasure of doing it well, those fleeting moments when time stills and my brain locks in and I ride an invisible wave that will leave me, an hour or a day later, tumbling alone toward the shore. Where did all that time I spent working go?

"It has to go somewhere," a writer friend reassures me gently. But what does she know? She sold her novel. She got away clean.

"Maybe you should try to write a television pilot," says a friend from my days as an assistant. She has grown up into a corporate lawyer at a white-shoe firm. Her husband is a TV and film agent and she says he will probably read it with an eye toward getting me a job. She adds tentatively, "Isn't it true that most artists are not very happy?"

COURTNEY, THE SOCIAL WORKER, SHOWS up at my mother's to deliver her Seroquel. My mother won't let her in because, as she explains, Hakeem Olajuwon told her she didn't have to. Courtney, as she's required to, calls in a wellness check. A training force comes and breaks down the door to my grandmother's office. My mother refuses to go to the hospital and drops out of the program on the spot. The county is not, by law, allowed to force a patient to take medication if they don't want to. And so she is back to where she started and there is nothing any of us can do.

...

JILL WRITES TO SAY SHE has bad news, then calls me. She's sorry, she says. She made a mistake. The short of it is, upon finishing this draft, she doesn't think the book is quite there yet. It needs more work before she can submit. She wonders if there is an Afrofuturism thread to be included. Have I seen the film *Sorry to Bother You*? What she's saying without saying it is that for the book to sell, it needs to be Blacker. It's not the fault of the book or the writer—only the zeitgeist. I don't blame her for telling me this. She's only doing her job. I nod into the phone and write down her notes and, when the call is over, make my way to the French restaurant on the corner where we had our first meeting and get drunk at a table outside by myself. I think about all the people who have written and sold books over the course of the history of the world. It never seemed possible that every single one of these people was smarter and harder-working than me. But maybe they were. Maybe this is a mercy killing. Maybe all I needed was for someone to come along and finally put this project out of its misery.

I text Ethan but he's out with his intern auditioning actors for a new film. I go home and sit alone at my desk in my bedroom for a while. *You're okay. You're okay. You're okay*, I think.

IN 1938, WALTER BENJAMIN FASHIONED a long essay out of the notes that would become *The Arcades Project*, centered on the work of the poet Charles Baudelaire. He turned the essay in to its commissioning body later that year and it was swiftly rejected. His friend and editor Theodor Adorno called the work "a wide-eyed presentation of mere facticity . . . consumed in its own aura" and stuck "at the . . . 'crossroads of magic and positivism.'"[34]

Benjamin's devastation was total. The essay was the culmination of his life's work, and its publication was also all he had to rely on for income. The dismissal of his efforts as "abstract theorizing," coming at a time when Benjamin was almost entirely without resources, led him to write letters that alarmed his friends and to disappear from public life for months.[35] Two years later, he would be dead and the Arcades Project would remain incomplete. "Even if Benjamin had lived long enough," writes critic and poet Adam Kirsch, "it is doubtful that he could have completed it."[36] Thanks to Adorno's crushing response, "The intellectual and ideological basis of the work was in ruins."

In 2018, I throw my laptop across the room. I hear a crack as its protective case splits. The sound is satisfying, but I still can't feel anything, and I want to feel something. And so a clay mug Ethan brought home from Estonia that I've been using as a pencil holder follows my laptop in its arc through the air. Then a glass paperweight in the shape of a globe, then a set of three small IKEA drawers housing all my 1099s from the past several years. Cheaply made, it shatters on impact with the ground.

Then a folder full of college work: copies of poems by Catullus, notes on Rilke's letters to Rodin, essays on Apollo versus Dionysus, then every journal I filled in New York and every note I made for my novel in the notepads I stole from every office job I ever had, then a plastic warthog a novelist gave me once when I took a summer workshop she taught ("If you ever decide to give up on your novel," she said, passing the little animals around the room, "do me a favor and throw this guy away," the idea being that the animals were cute enough that we would never throw them away and thus we would never give up on our books), and a plastic bumblebee my friend Lydia gave me at a residency in Virginia, and every draft of *The Anatomy Book*, every acceptance letter and graduation photograph and every postcard I ever received and book after book after book from the shelves above my desk, all land in a pile in front of my bedroom door, trapping me inside.

I empty a second standing bookshelf into the pile. Goodbye *Open City* and *The Association of Small Bombs* and *Fates and Furies* and *Fortune Smiles* and *The Turner House* and *Delicious Foods* and *The Sympathizer* and *The Beautiful Bureaucrat* and *A Constellation of Vital Phenomena* and *A Visit from the Goon Squad* and *Battleborn*. Farewell also *Drown* and *Birds of America* and *The Emigrants* and *Play It as It Lays* and *Life on Mars* and *War and Peace* and *Illuminations* and *The Golden Compass* and *The Collected Stories of Lydia Davis* and *The Moviegoer* and *Vertigo* and *Dubliners* and *Portrait of the Artist as a Young Man* and *Remainder* and *Pnin* and *The Journalist and the Murderer* and *Man Walks into a Room* and *The End of the Story* and *On Writing*. For so long, I looked at the world through the lens of fiction, but now that lens is gone and reality rushes back in startling color. And even while it's happening I am resisting the urge to narrate it. I'm so terribly sick of cannibalizing myself for art, writing short stories about women who are like me but are not me and whose mothers are far away or do not exist. Always on the lookout for anything in the real world that can be dragged into the narrative one and exploited. Always separate from my own life so I can witness and describe it. My head empties as I scrabble over the pile and out of my bedroom through the front door carrying an armful of books and papers, sweating. My brain feels like a broken spring, ping-ponging this way and that.

Throwing away the books means throwing away the time my novel has taken from me, means throwing away the jobs I didn't apply for, the friends I lost or didn't make, the phone calls I didn't place to my mother, Sadie, all of my unachievable dreams. I don't know how to neutralize this pain but I know how to make it worse, and in this way remain in control.

"You know what I think? I think you want to be crazy," my college boyfriend once said to me, mid-breakup. "Because then you wouldn't have to do anything." It was the meanest thing this person ever said about me but perhaps also the most accurate, and I remember holding the statement up and studying its light from every angle, then storing it away in a dark place. Here now is proof that he was right. It feels good to give in. To let the world divide along its cracks and fall to pieces with it. No one told me how much better it would feel to destroy than to create, to throw everything I love away so I can't lose it.

I run back into my bedroom to gather more papers and books from the pile. I hear the front door open. Ethan coming home. Before he can say anything I scurry down the hallway into the bathroom to hide. I peel my clothes off and step into the shower so that it won't be obvious what I'm doing, which is hiding in the only room in our apartment with a lock. But when I come out wrapped in a towel, I find the dog sitting outside with her tail between her legs, Ethan waving a broken shard of Estonian mug at me like an accusation.

"You threw away your Kafka? Your Sebald?" Ethan surveys the damage I've done to my bookshelves. "Do I need to take you somewhere?" he asks, lips set in a thin line.

I lie flat on my back on the bed. I still feel as if I am floating outside myself, but the feeling is not unpleasant. "This is a good thing," I say, only half-disingenuously. "I'm making room for something new."

"How would you feel if you came home one afternoon and every DVD I owned was gone? My camera equipment?"

I tell him to stop being so dramatic. He tells me to stop throwing tantrums like a child. When I laugh at him, he throws Jay-Z's autobiography, which he got me for my birthday years ago and has retrieved from a garbage can out back, onto the floor. The dog hides under the bed in fear and peeks out at us, shaking, and we both find ourselves on our knees, apologizing to her and begging her to come out.

I can tell Ethan is afraid this outburst is the first small step toward my following in my mother's footsteps. I don't know how to explain to him that now that I have decided to throw myself into the void I've spent my whole life sidestepping, it turns out it wasn't actually there. The pain that I wanted to rip my consciousness to pieces did not. The world went on and nothing changed. I kick back through the pile of objects spread out across the bedroom floor and burst into the hallway.

"If you do this again, I'm leaving you," Ethan says, following me. And though he sounds angry, I know he's afraid. This is not what he signed up for. He lives for order. He gets annoyed when I drop my coat over the edge of the couch instead of hanging it up or when I kick off my shoes by the door and leave them there. You would be the perfect girlfriend if you could remember to wash your dishes, he grumbles at me sometimes from the kitchen, scrubbing the half-empty coffee mugs I've abandoned in every room.

"Then leave me," I say, not a threat or a challenge but possibly a demand for the most logical outcome to finally occur, for him to follow through on the inevitable.

"You're trying to hurt yourself. The opposite of what Sadie does. She hurts other people and you hurt yourself. But it's the same thing."

"Stop yelling," I say to Ethan. "I can hear you."

I don't believe I'm going to actually marry Ethan, not because I don't want to but because I don't believe anything good that happens to me can last. Even when I imagine our wedding, it doesn't feel real. If asked what I thought a real future for the two of us might look like, the answer I would give wouldn't involve marriage at all but some kind of long-term affair in which he marries someone more suitable and I work in a faraway city and we write emails and see each other occasionally. The one essential thing is that he always be somewhere in the world for me to find. So it seems only natural to me now that he, too, would go.

I ask him if I can go to sleep. Just this one time, I implore, can we not talk? To my surprise, he agrees, retreating into a silence that is foreign to our household but not to me. I fall asleep alone in our bed imagining what will happen when I wake up and Ethan is gone and I have to start the process of figuring out how to escape it again.

But I wake up in the morning to discover that not only has

Ethan not left, he has quietly pulled my books out of the trash. On the DVD shelves in the living room are my essay collections by Baldwin, my plays by Sarah Ruhl, my popular science books by Brian Greene, and my novels by W. G. Sebald. Here is the paper on Kafka by my favorite grad school professor. Here is an anthology of writing about California with my name on the cover because I edited it. Here are the literary journals my work appears in. He's rescued as much of what I threw out as he could, and though he could not retrieve it all, he has retrieved those books he knew I would miss the most. I'd read and annotated Kafka's journals the summer after I graduated from NYU. Not only would they have been gone, the notes I'd made and the memories I associated with the hours I'd spent reading them—the readness of them—would have been gone too. Now here they are, back in the apartment, on Ethan's shelves instead of mine.

That day, books keep surfacing in the backyard, rescued by well-meaning neighbors and the people who go through the trash for recyclables at night. *Nine Stories* and *My Life as a Man* and *On Beauty* and *The Immigrants* and *The Bluest Eye* and *A Moveable Feast*. They assemble on the sidewalk in front of our building, seem to be trying to find their way inside. I ignore them. And when I am not home, Ethan picks them up and brings them, one by one, back into the house. He instructs me not to touch them. Says they belong to him now, and I am not to throw away his things.

THIRTEEN

ETHAN AND I DRIVE TO San Francisco for Fourth of July weekend. A cousin of his, a partner at a corporate law firm, is always traveling for work and has an empty apartment in Russian Hill. Ethan lets me choose everything we do, even if it's cheesy or we've done it before. We walk down Lombard Street. We go to a coffee shop the size of an airplane hangar. We eat vegan Vietnamese sandwiches on the sidewalk. Without the manuscript haunting my thoughts, I move from place to place in a kind of blank wonder. What was I hiding from in my novel? Why did I feel the need to hide from it for so long? And now that I've stepped out from behind it, will whatever it was finally find me?

"Are you going to write something new?" Ethan asks.

"No," I say. "That would be insane."

Ethan sighs. He is furious with me for giving up, but scared of what I'll do if he shows it.

"Do you think—" he asks.

"Think what?"

"Do you think maybe you should call your dad?"

The idea shocks me out of my spiral of self-pity, if only because it makes no sense. I speak to my dad maybe once every two years.

He's the only person I know who at any given moment is guaranteed to be worse off than I am. But when I search for actual reasons not to call him, I can't find any. It's true that my mother may forget me soon. It's probably in my best interest to have at least one of my parents know that I exist and care that I'm alive.

I send him a text and he calls back right away. He doesn't sound surprised to hear from me. He lives in a state of perpetual hope. Years ago, he took the Foreign Service exam without studying, then seemed surprised when he failed. He drinks too much and smokes too much and yet he may be my happiest relative, still calls my grandmother from time to time to check in and keep her updated on his life, which delights her.

We make a plan to meet at Lake Merritt. When Ethan and I arrive, we sit on the grass by the water, watching the dog sniff some leaves. I check the time on my phone. "What if he was here already and he left?"

"No offense," Ethan says, "but your dad doesn't strike me as the kind of person who shows up when he says he will."

We make our way to a coffee shop, where I get a too-sweet Italian soda and Ethan gets an espresso and we both get toasted bagels with plain hummus. We find a bench to sit on, and then I leave to use the bathroom at a restaurant on the water. The dog tries to follow me inside and cries when she can't.

I come out of the restaurant as my dad appears, thirty minutes late, loping through the tall grass down to the bench where Ethan is. The first thing I see is that he is missing his two front teeth. I stare at the blank spaces. He puts a hand over his mouth, demure, and says, "You're looking at my teeth."

"What happened?"

"I fell down," he says.

"Did someone push you?" I ask. He shakes his head. He was coming from his favorite barbecue joint, where he'd gone to drink beer and dance, he says. He was walking back home with a bag of chicken in his hand, and the next thing he knew he was waking up in the hospital, having fallen face-first.

"Is that how you got those bruises?" I ask him. Thin black lines trace curves down his forehead and his cheekbones. No, he says, but does not elaborate, and I don't ask again. Later, I'll learn from one of his sisters that he didn't fall at all, that someone beat him up and robbed him outside a bar.

I pat my pockets and search through my purse. "I can't find my phone," I say. And indeed my phone is gone. I retrace my steps to the bathroom of the fancy restaurant, but it isn't there. Relief washes over me. I'm free. I can run away from this meeting, from myself, change my name, start a new life, no longer be addicted to a thing that makes me sad. But when I walk outside, a waiter recognizes me from the picture with Ethan and the dog I use as wallpaper and pushes the found device toward me. I accept it with a mix of gratitude and reluctance, briefly wishing I had the courage to fling it into the lake.

When I return, I can tell Ethan and my dad have become friends. The only other time they've met was at my cousin's wedding, and this is the first time they've been alone together. Ethan is telling him a story but he stops talking when I approach.

"What?" I say, suspicious.

"Nothing," my dad says, gazing out over the smooth water. He offers Ethan a sidelong glance. This is what my dad does, makes everyone feel as if being near him means being in on a very important secret. It is obvious Ethan told him we are engaged, but I don't say anything. I don't want to ruin their little moment.

"How did you and my mom meet?" I ask instead.

"I was a sophomore at San Francisco State University. I was studying Rastafarianism and growing out my hair and learning the many hidden histories of ancient Africa, Ethiopian Orthodoxy, and ancient Hebrew kings," he says. "Eating natural foods and being separate from the Babylon system. I worked on campus driving a golf cart. One day on my route, I passed by the most beautiful girl I had ever seen."

When he saw her again later at a juice stand where he also worked, he asked for her number, but she had a boyfriend. "The boyfriend had been on a team I played basketball against in high school. We were the winningest basketball team in the history of the state at that time!"

He pauses, as if for applause, and, when I don't react, continues his story. He took my mother back to his apartment to make popcorn, then to meet his family at his parents' house on Holly Street, in Oakland. She was the first girl he ever brought home.

"We got married on March twenty-first, nineteen eighty-five, at an exclusive private wedding event at Knowland Park in Oakland Hills. We moved to an apartment near Park Boulevard, which we rented from a Portuguese woman named Mrs. Siena, who charged us three hundred seventy-five dollars a month. She was very wise." But, my dad says solemnly, he knew my mother was sad. She kept a journal about her father, whose death she thought was probably a hit job.

"Your grandfather was a baller, and many people wanted him dead," he says. "Eventually your grandmother made your mother come back to Houston. I cried and cried. I was working three jobs and we had two cars and a nice apartment. I finished college at San Francisco State and went to Houston to visit you twice a year."

His version seems to be missing a section, or many sections. In my mother's telling, my dad had zero jobs, not three, and according to her it was he who told her to leave with me and not come back. "If I could get through that," she once said about their marriage, "then I could get through anything."

I tell him about the voices she hears, her paranoia, her anger. That she lost her job and lives in my grandmother's office because she can't afford to pay rent.

"She's always been like that," he says.

"She heard voices?"

"Sort of. She used to make up conflicts that didn't exist."

"Well, it certainly would have been nice if someone had mentioned that to me," I say, sitting down on the bench. I say it as though I am exasperated with my dad, when really, I am exasperated by the patterns that keep resurfacing, and my own inability to answer the questions they pose: At what point does habitual anger become madness? Where is the dividing line between someone who is always furious and someone who is psychotic? What is the difference between my mother's rage, which is irrational; Sadie's, which sometimes feels rational; and my own, which I can hardly feel at all but which I sometimes suspect secretly drives everything I do? Is it really a matter of degree? I look around for the rest of my bagel. Ethan shrugs when I can't find it.

"The dog," he says, and Larry Bird gazes up at me, serene, with hummus on her nose.

"Thanks," I snap at both of them. "Thank you for letting the dog eat my bagel."

"I can go to Houston and take care of her," my dad says then. "Your mom, I mean. You said she lost her job. She doesn't have any money. She's in and out of the hospital. She needs somebody."

"I'll ask her what she thinks," I say.

"I just read a novel," he tells me then. "*A Lesson Before Dying*, by Ernest J. Gaines." The book is set in Bayonne, Louisiana, a fictional town not unlike the one where his father—my grandfather—was from. A difficult place for a Black man in the forties, he says. "You had a house and you had food, but you couldn't get a good education. Or a good job. That does something to you. It made me think . . . I'm one generation removed from there, so my faults . . . some of it is . . . I inherited it, really."

What about what I inherited? I think, angry. He's trying to give me the explanation he thinks I want, but I don't want it from him. I listen to the cars whirring behind us on the road until my dad stands up and brushes off his pants, unperturbed by my silence. "You should probably visit your sister," he says. "I told her you two were here."

My dad has two daughters by his second wife, Joelle and Tiffany, my half sisters. They are easygoing, pretty girls in their early twenties who were popular in high school and who grew up feeling more emotionally bonded to him than I do, even though he left them and their mother, too, when they were very young. The younger of the two, Joelle, now has a little girl of her own. They live with her grandmother in a suburb outside Oakland in a house at the top of a hill. My sisters' people on their mom's side are from Cameron, Louisiana, and they inherited the beige skin and wavy hair endemic to that region. "Look, I've been out in the sun, so I look dark like you!" they would say to me when they were younger, holding up their skinny yellow arms to my brown ones so we could compare.

Now my dad hugs us goodbye, and I watch him walk away in the direction of the BART station. We drive to San Leandro, where Joelle lives. While Ethan lights up the grill and she makes guacamole, I sit with her almost two-year-old daughter and help her build stacks of hollow blocks and knock them down again. Larry Bird pokes around at first terrifying, then delighting, the baby, who tries to stick her hands inside the dog's mouth. Ethan rescues the dog by lifting the baby up on his shoulders and taking her out onto the back porch to see the Fourth of July fireworks barely visible above the skyline.

Joelle's grandmother and mother and her mother's boyfriend watch TV in the living room. I listen to the sleepy buzz of their voices, the clink of beer bottles against the coffee table. In the kitchen, my sister sips from a glass of water and pours me syrupy white wine. She is more grown-up now that she has the baby. Something in her face makes her seem older than me, all traces of the high school cheerleader she was subsumed by this person who knows things. She asks me how I've been. I consider telling the truth about my mother, about how I worry she is going to step out into traffic and die or wander off or hurt someone in my family. But I can imagine, all the time I am talking, my sister's face growing more and more upset. The point would be to forge a connection but instead I will feel hollowed out and empty, my story cheapened because I told it. Pity will turn it into a block of stone inside my body that I will never be able to carve out, and I don't want this hurt to calcify, don't want to forget how quickly everything can change. So we make small talk about the baby and the fireworks, and her ex, who lives nearby, and then Ethan and I drive back to the apartment in Russian Hill. The whole time we are driving, I am thinking that although I love my sister and I want to love my dad, I am not in the right city.

FOURTEEN

AS SOON AS WE GET back to Los Angeles, I leave Ethan and the dog and fly to Houston. On a layover at SFO, I buy a coffee and a Vietnamese sandwich and then I buy my mother a copy of Tayari Jones's *An American Marriage*, though I don't know whether she will be lucid enough to read it. I fly into Houston at sunset, watch the city bleed up through the clouds in squares, a life-sized map of itself. I search for buildings I recognize, but in the dusk, the whole city looks foreign.

My mother calls me almost the second I land to ask if my flight was okay, how I am doing, and then she asks the same questions again in a way that signals she doesn't want to let me off the phone.

"Are you here?

"How was your flight?

"How is the dog?

"How is Ethan?

"How was your flight?

"How is Ethan?

"How is the dog?

"How was your flight?"

When I tell her I have to go, she says, "I'll stay on the phone with you until you get a cab."

She is afraid I will take a rideshare and wind up raped and murdered in an alley somewhere by Lance Blanks. I am furious with a teenager's fury—I feel myself regressing to a thirteen-year-old version of myself enraged at not being allowed to go to a friend's house because my mother assumed there would be drugs, even though my friends and I weren't cool enough to ever have been offered any.

Families and women pushing baby carriages and flight attendants gathering their luggage stream past me out of the airport and into the night. "I have to get off the phone to get a cab," I tell my mother, my voice lilting upwards into a screech the way it did when I was young and I wanted her to leave me alone. "I'm an adult. I have my own apartment. I live in Los Angeles. You're driving me a little bit crazy. I need you to let me go get a ride so I can get home." Home for the night is the apartment where we lived when I was little in the fourplex my grandmother owns, now between tenants. My mother will also be in the same complex, in the rooms just below that were once part of my grandmother's office.

On the phone, she's laughing at me, and I'm shouting at her that it's not funny, but it is a little funny, and I think if I can still be angry with her, if we can still argue the way we did when I was young, then both of us might be okay. I tell her I'm getting into a taxi, then summon a Lyft, and half an hour later, I am in bed at the old apartment.

IN THE MORNING, AFTER I brush my teeth and wash my face and get dressed, I text my mother, but she doesn't respond. It's early August, and I wander outside into a thick, swampy heat that feels like both a blanket and a welcome. Cicada shells piled up on sidewalks like prehistoric monsters startle me before I remember they're harmless, only skin. I pass the crepe myrtle trees whose buds I used to squeeze open with my fingers, an eight-year-old's act of wanton destruction. I feel glad the trees are taller now, their branches safely beyond my reach.

At 9:00 a.m. it is already extraordinarily hot. I duck into a church parking lot with a wall around it to slip my bra off over my head and stuff it in my purse. The church has the same blue brick walls as the pool where I took swimming lessons. When I lived here back when I was very young, I thought the church and the pool were the same building, even though they were on opposite sides of town.

At first, I worry I've forgotten how to make eye contact, how to wave and say hello to strangers—this is not something people do in Los Angeles—but after the third person I pass, it becomes second nature again. A boy walks by with a German shepherd on a leash and steps off the sidewalk so I can go past. A second woman walks by with two schnauzers. I keep expecting giant stray dogs to rear up out of nowhere the way they used to when I was little and the neighborhood was a different place, a place where nobody walked.

When I check my phone, I discover that, according to Google Maps, this area is now called the Museum District—an effort, I guess, to attract the kinds of homebuyers who don't want to live in a place called Third Ward. I put my phone back in my pocket and pass a row of ugly town houses that look like Lego blocks, wildly out of place between the big old brick mansions, haunted-looking and mossy, that border them on either side.

On Almeda, I go into a strip mall coffee shop called Kaffeine and am surprised to find a pecan-colored woman with a head wrap and a gold tooth behind the counter. Black people didn't own coffee shops in the Third Ward I used to know, because there were no coffee shops here when I was young. The seats inside are filled with a mix of Black and white, young and old. I sit down beside two men on a date. One of the men is slim and attractive, and I am struck by the unequal power dynamic between him and his counterpart, a bumbling, blushing man with an Irish accent wearing red suspenders. The date is not going well. The Irish man keeps asking questions, but the slender boy asks none. The suspender-wearing man's voice grows loud with desperation: "Maybe the world ended in 2012, like the Mayans predicted, and this is what it looks like"—a joke about the state of the world after Trump's election that the slim boy doesn't seem to understand. I get the uncanny feeling I'm in two places at once, both here and down the street from my apartment in Los Feliz, eavesdropping on two hipsters who met on a dating app. I leave, taking my iced coffee with me out into the hot day.

And suddenly I'm in Houston again, with the sky too big and nothing to temper the massive clouds that arch across the ground, beckoning me into another world. I forgot what it was like to stand in one spot on a wide, flat road and see the entire city, and I wait there, awestruck, in a crosswalk long after the light turns. A man in a pickup truck honks at me. "Hey, skinny girl!" he calls out as he speeds off, and then it is twenty years ago and I am thirteen and he is the old man whistling at me from a passing Impala, shouting, "Hey, high-yaller girl!" making my mother laugh as we come out of the you-buy-we-fry fish place that used to sit on this corner but doesn't anymore. My mother repeated the man's phrase "hey, high-yaller" softly, liking the way it sounded. I reach for that moment layered somewhere under this one, buried, not gone, but impossible to touch.

Here is the Walgreens where I once saw a man dressed like Jesus ask the cashier for cigarettes. When she bent behind the register to retrieve them, he ran out of the store with his arms full of stolen batteries, candy bars, and gum. ("That man took all that stuff," the cashier said to me, mystified, blinking long, false eyelashes lined with crystals.) Here is the Reggae Hut, with its delicious rice and peas and terrible service. Here is Lee's Nails, where my mother took me to get my eyebrows waxed for the first time when I was twelve. Here is the African beauty supply shop, where she bought the shea butter she combed through her hair on weekends. I text my mother again, then call her, and she doesn't respond. I wonder if the argument we had on the phone last night was more significant than I thought. If, in the time from then to now, she's gone from being concerned to enraged with me, which is something that happens a lot.

When I was very young, we were constantly chasing each other, my mother coming on too strong and me, irritated, pulling away, which led her to shut me out completely, which led me to chase her again. Later I could wallow for days in the blue moods that came over me when she would not speak to me, refusing to answer the phone when I called, leaving me behind like something rejected and diseased. Her silence sat on my chest and infected everything around me, until I did the same thing to her, ignoring her calls out of a desire to prevent her from hurting me again. Then I did the same to Sadie. Is the rest of my life going to be like this? Am I going to spend it hiding from other people's anger and my own?

My mother is in her rooms at the office with the shades pulled down when I go to visit her that afternoon. She opens the glass-paned front door before I can knock. It turns out she has not been ignoring me. She had her phone off all day because the voices in her head have been plaguing her. I can see the tension in her face now as she tries to ignore them.

"I made you some lunch," she says, and gestures at a peanut butter and jelly sandwich and a banana and an apple and a kiwi. This small act, peanut butter spread on Wonder Bread sliced in half and placed in a Ziploc bag, neatly undoes me. I once thought the trauma in my family served simply as an obstacle I had to overcome to achieve greatness. Remembering this now, I swallow the bile that rises in my throat. She crosses the room and retrieves a cup of muddy brown liquid, which she hands to me. "I made you some molasses tea," she says. "It's good for you, cleans you right out." She has warmed the tea up on a metal space heater in the corner, which she turned on, presumably to cook with, even though it is almost 100 degrees outside. Something is growing in a speckled black pattern across the painted windowsill that looks out onto the front yard. It gives the room a fetid smell. We move into the second room, where my mother keeps a small flat mattress on the floor, next to a box of what looks like dried leaves.

I ask her about the box. She tells me she was starved for eight

187

days by my grandmother and Aunt Tina. She ate dandelions, soaking them in hot water to cook. She believes the food they brought her was tainted. I ask her if the thoughts go away when she takes her meds. She reminds me that Hakeem Olajuwon said she doesn't have to take her medication anymore.

I think, If the patterns I saw in Paris meant what I thought they did, if everything that grows is shaped like a branching tree, and if the core of that shape is the trunk that runs through it, then life itself is that trunk, and all of us are branches, elements of a process of death and rebirth that progresses along a continuum we will never be able to see. Both of us, my mother and I, are a step toward something new and our lives are part of something bigger, something flawed but changing.

I wipe down the mildewed surfaces and empty the containers of rotting oatmeal and straighten up the books and take my mother's dirty clothes down to the washing machine in the basement and open the windows so air can come in, and then I clean her pencil drawings off the walls with a damp cloth and cleaning spray. She watches me, wary, her voice caught in loops—"I'm so sorry, Sarah, I'm just talking"—the story of Lance's harassment coming out of her over and over in waves.

"If I try to go outside right now, other people will come out and walk real fast in front of me. They pretend to have conversations. They just materialize in front of me. I try to go to church, and Lance has gotten to the pastor, so I can tell nothing he's saying is real. They push the collection plate in my face like they can tell I don't have anything to put in it. I went to a different church. Lance followed me there, so I stopped trying. It was a waste of my time."

She points to cracks in the wall, tells me they are Lance attempting to communicate with her in secret messages only she can interpret. "He puts these here to remind me," she says.

Outside, I gulp fresh air like water and sob a little, then call Ethan, who makes comforting noises in the form of words I can't comprehend. I am remembering a night when I was seven years old, and my mother left me at home alone to go for a jog around the neighborhood. I ran out of the apartment into the street in a panic, because I didn't know where she was. I fell and scraped my knees on the sidewalk. When she heard me crying, she came running back, shouting and angry because I needed her so badly, because she could never do anything alone. Though years have passed, the fear in my heart that she is gone forever and I've been left behind remains. I will get over the loss of Sadie, since when a friend says you're no longer friends, then you're no longer friends, but there is nothing my mother or I can say that will stop her from being my mother, and where she's run away to is not a physical place, and so I cannot chase her there or convince her to run back to me.

I WALK UNTIL I GET to the Museum of Fine Arts, which, on summer Thursdays, stays open late, plays music and has cheap wine on offer at kiosks outside. I order a glass of sauvignon blanc and join a crowd of strangers who listen to a docent explain how Renaissance painters created shadows: not as individual images, she says, but with a wash, a kind of filter that turned parts of the canvas green-gray.

I nod along, only able to think of ways in which these shadows are a metaphor for what my mother's disorder is doing to her, enveloping her and then shadowing her completely, then tune out the docent to focus on the Nina Simone song playing from the museum speakers and the pain in Nina's voice:

I'm gonna leave you yes I'm gonna
I'm gonna leave you cos I wanna
And I'll go where people love me
And I'll stay there cos they love me.

I know she is talking about her husband, who beat her, and her daughter, whom she drove away. I think about how Simone's bipolar behavior was never diagnosed or medicated. She spent the second half of her life fleeing the disorder and was never cured.

IN THE MORNING, MY GRANDMOTHER picks me up to take me to see her city garden plot near the freeway. On the drive, she tells me stories about people I knew when I was growing up, like the man from St. Thomas, Winston, an ex of my mother's whom she met at my grandmother's office when he was a patient. He brought me vintage pins with sayings on them like "Don't laugh! I'm making a fashion statement!" and invited all his noisy cousins over for parties. He made fun of my mother when she fussed at me, which briefly turned our lives sunny. He remained a family friend even after they broke up, and later went to prison for dealing marijuana. Before he went in, he married his girlfriend, a Cameroonian royal who managed his money for him. When he got out, my grand-mother tells me, he was rich. "He opened a big-rig repair business and they had three kids, the third one born with severe develop-mental delays," she reports.

Another friend of my grandmother's, Patrice, a Vietnam vet who lives in a garage, was diagnosed with cancer and then told he didn't have it—because, my grandmother suspects, his insurance wasn't good enough to cover continued treatments. "But the thing is, he believes he doesn't have it, even though I think they didn't want to treat him anymore. And miraculously, he looks much bet-ter now!" she confides. "He gained all his weight back. His skin had turned yellow. Now it's brown again." She points out the giant okra vines in her garden plot, the eggplant and peppers growing in the shade, the smokers some of the neighborhood men will haul out later in the evening to drink around. The lemongrass and cit-rus trees and kale, all green and sturdy in the sunlight.

We go to the farmers' market on Bagby for lunch, and she runs her fingers across the hard speckled pears and muscadine grapes, exclaims over a truck full of watermelon, buys a baby fig tree for ten dollars, and tells me sadly about the plants my mother dug up and threw at her when she tried to keep a garden patch behind her office. Because I ask her to, she drives me to the psychiatric hospi-tal where my mother is occasionally an inpatient.

"When she got mad at me, she used to say she was going to bring me here and have me committed and the doctors were going to shove pills down my throat until I choked," I hear myself say out loud. My grandmother looks stricken.

"I didn't know that," she says.

191

Of course she didn't. But at that age I still thought Aunt Tina and my grandmother and my mother knew everything. Down the street from the psychiatric hospital sits the house in Riverside Terrace. We drive there and park out front. In the distance I hear the cars on Highway 288, which runs directly through the center of this mostly Black neighborhood, a reminder that even though the houses are big and pretty and well constructed, that wasn't enough to stop city planners from deciding they mattered little enough to destroy. The problem isn't us, I think. It's what already happened. It's pain layered over itself until it became my mother's illness, my distance and indifference, and everything else for which we cannot forgive ourselves, even though it's not our fault.

THAT NIGHT I GO OUT with Aunt Tina and her best friend, Venita, to a happy hour off Westheimer, near the Galleria. At the bar, I drink grapefruit juice and vodka and eat French fries while my aunt and Venita flirt with the bartender, who looks like Donald Glover and has a broken arm. The air-conditioning is up so high it gets into my bones—these aggressive HVAC systems, too, are something I forget about every time I leave, am only remembering now that I am home. I ask Aunt Tina if she misses my mother, the good parts of her, at least.

"I never had the good parts," she says. "I didn't know there were good parts. She was always mean or ignoring me. It's just the way she was."

I need her to know there were good parts. That I got the good parts. The parts no one else got to have. "Once," I say, "she took me to a Black ski club meeting even though neither one of us ever skied. We didn't even own skis. I still haven't gone skiing."

"A Black ski club? In Houston?" Aunt Tina pulls a face. "Are you sure that's right?"

I pull my phone out and search "Black ski club, Houston," and there it is, the Ski Jammers, a group devoted to supporting the activities of Black skiers and snowboarders. No experience necessary. She wanted me to have a life that didn't look like hers, and that is why I have the life I have. Because she imagined a new world for us, no matter how strange, and refused to let the idea of it go.

Aunt Tina and Venita finish their drinks and want to go to the Davenport, a dive bar on Richmond, to dance with the old barflies, but my aunt is eyeing me, looking worried. I ordered a second Greyhound when she got up to go to the bathroom and drank it quickly, finishing it before she came back, so I could order a third, but I was not expecting her to grab the bill and pay it when it came. She knows I had three drinks, not two, and that I finished the middle one secretly.

"I don't think Sarah should drink anymore," she says.

"Oh." Now Venita looks at me critically too. "Then you need to be dropped off at home."

I let them drop me at the old apartment, and then, once they're gone, I take a Lyft alone to a bar on Westheimer that I find by searching Yelp. Outside the bar, I find a crowd of well-dressed Black people who all seem to be regulars and who can tell I am not one. It is briefly jarring to be around so many people who look like me when my neighborhood in Los Angeles—and everywhere I go in Los Angeles, really—feels monochrome in a way I've grown used to against my will.

The sidewalk is crowded with tables, and the entryway isn't visible from the street. After three sweeps past the fashionable crowd looking for the front door while trying not to make it look like that is what I am doing, I give up and go to the James Coney Island hot dog place across the street to order fries. When I get there the door is locked, and then I am alone in the dark on a concrete island in the middle of the city.

Sober now, I remember Houston is not a pedestrian-friendly city, especially not at night, especially when the pedestrian doesn't know where they are going or where they are, is lost in a place they once knew as well as they knew anything. I can call another Lyft, but I don't know where to ask it to take me. Google Maps is no help, and the truth is I don't want it to be. I want to know where I am instinctively, the way I would have fifteen years ago, when I would have remembered that it doesn't make sense to try to navigate this part of the city on foot. I think of my mother walking along C. E. King Parkway. Panic blooms. To quell it, I walk down the sidewalk, headed nowhere now.

I make my way down Richmond, past liquor stores and a fancy new Starbucks and a storage center that takes up half a block, and then I am facing La Tapatia, the Mexican restaurant I used to come to with my high school best friend, Amy, because the servers would bring us margaritas without asking for ID. Where once it took up only the corner of a strip mall, now it is huge, with a garden patio, and has swallowed up the laundromat and convenience store next to it like an amoeba. I sit down at a table outside and order two tacos, rice, beans, guacamole, and a margarita—I don't know what else to do, and, waiting, I am seventeen again with Amy, who stopped speaking to me after we tried to live together in Los Angeles after college and fell out over her then-boyfriend, a coke-dealer fifteen years our senior. Amy is here, across the table laughing at me for being so sad, and then she is gone and I am by myself at a Mexican restaurant in my home city, in my thirties, still not having published a novel or made any money, and merengue music plays while high schoolers drinking margaritas for which they have not been carded glance at me and wonder who the sad woman is drinking alone. Or they don't wonder that, because they don't see me—they look past me, the way I looked past anybody at that age I didn't want to befriend or sleep with. By the time the waitress brings my order, I don't want it anymore, because Houston is the saddest city and all I want is to go home to my life in L.A. or go back to my life here when I was a teenager, eating tacos with Amy. Enjoy it while you can, I think of saying to the table of high schoolers with their bright, ill-gotten drinks, and then I take back the thought. Maybe knowing you are supposed to enjoy something makes it impossible to enjoy that thing. Enjoy it because you can, I think. Enjoy it because it's yours.

I call a Lyft to come get me and then I am back in Third Ward, alone at night, the houses looming over me in the dark. I sit outside my grandmother's office on the porch and listen to my mother's gospel music play loudly through the window, Eddie Levert's low, heavy voice backed by a choir—*Thank you, thank you, thank you, thank you*, the choir sings again and again. *Thank you. Thank you. Thank you.* I climb the steps and stop at the door of my mother's room and she opens it wide, as if she has been expecting me. She sits back down in her desk chair and I watch her sway from side to side and sing. I search her face for a sign of the woman who raised me, buried embers softly glowing. From a certain angle in the low-lit room, I can almost see her. From another, I can see my grandmother and from another, myself. I breathe on the flames, fan them with my mind, will them not to burn out, try to send them strength to grow.

FIFTEEN

IT'S SEPTEMBER 2019, THE MONTH before Ethan and I get married. Ethan, in pre-production on a film in Guatemala, calls me between meetings to go over seating charts, alcohol, hotel blocks. We fight with the very traditional wedding planner about our right to a vegetarian menu. We fight with each other about a wooden salad bowl I want to add to the registry that Ethan keeps calling "pointless." By the time the week of the ceremony arrives, I feel as if we've already wed and divorced several times.

The day before we leave for Ted and Diana's ranch, I go to a final fitting in Glendale and get so physically ill I have to rip my wedding dress off and run to the bathroom, barely making it in time. I sleep for the next twelve hours while Ethan calls a friend to pick up my dress and pack the car and attends the final rehearsal for our first dance alone, with the male choreographer we hired standing in as me. I sleep more on the three-hour ride up to the ranch in Paso Robles, and when I arrive, our wedding planner invites a nurse over to hook me up to an intravenous vitamin drip.

I wake up feeling incredible and spend the afternoon alone in a strip mall Chinese restaurant wearing a fake fur coat I bought special for this weekend, eating noodles and nursing glass after glass of wine. When the waitress delivers my fortune cookie and I open it and discover it is empty—that somehow she has given me a fortune cookie without a fortune in it—I shriek and drop it on the table, where it breaks in half.

"Is everything okay?" the waitress comes back over to ask.

Is it? I don't know. I pay and leave. The car I call to take me to our venue gets lost on a farm nearby and not even Google Maps can help.

"I really thought you weren't coming," Ethan says, when I finally show up an hour late.

"And yet, I did!" I say.

But the rehearsal goes off without a hitch, as does the catered dinner we have at a golf club afterward. Some of our friends spend the night at the farmhouse and we stay up late playing pool. The next day at the ceremony, my grandmother and Aunt Tina walk me down the aisle, Ethan's mother reads a passage from *War and Peace* about Pierre's love for Natasha ("The happiness before him appeared so inconceivable that if only he could attain it, it would be the end of all things. Everything ended with that"[37]) and Aunt Tina reads the Benedetti poem Ethan gave me when he proposed. The dog sits positioned beside us on a wine barrel in a flower crown and falls asleep while we say our vows. *How does it feel to be married now?* the guests ask. They say, *Your vows made me cry*, and *thank you so much for having us*, and *the food was amazing*, and *you look so pretty*, and *you two make me want to get married again*. The photographer lines us up for pictures and it's all really nice, actually. I don't know why I was so afraid.

After the reception, someone tells me Sadie recently boycotted the wedding of a mutual friend from college because Mark was invited, and though it's been years since we've spoken, it's nice to know she still cares for me, because I still care for her, too.

SHORTLY AFTER THAT, AN EMAIL arrives in my inbox from Lance Blanks, and I wonder if I am finally hallucinating. He saw my wedding announcement in the *New York Times* and wanted to congratulate me. He knew my mom. She may have spoken about him? They had once been close. My heart drops into my knees. I ask if he will call me.

When we talk, I decide not to tell him my mother didn't attend my wedding, that she currently lives under the delusion that the world around her is a façade, that her real life is somewhere in Ethiopia, where she has an imaginary husband. That she does not believe my grandmother is her mother or that my aunt is her sister. That I'm scared soon she won't remember me, and that if my own mother doesn't remember me, it's as if I never happened. Instead we talk about his daughter who is getting married soon and his parents in Texas, whom he visits often, and I offer only vague details about my mother's ill-health.

He says he'll be in Los Angeles in April for work and that if I want to, he will sit with me and go over his correspondence with my mother and then will tell me everything I want to know. He is very sad to hear she isn't well. She was a gem of a person to him. He's always felt an inexplicable connection to her. In his lifetime, he says, he's met hundreds of people, and not one of them was like her. He doesn't know what to call the relationship they had other than to say that he loved her. When they were young, they drove to Galveston in the VW Rabbit she had then, he remembers, singing along to the radio. Lance and I make plans to talk again soon, and I hang up to walk the dog. Outside, the sun drops down behind the hills and the evening spreads out over our heads full of the light that carries us with it forever from one moment into the next.

I TAKE HENRY'S SUGGESTION AND write a television pilot. It's a character-driven half-hour comedy about a Black girl who loves her white fiancé but feels iffy about marriage and bribes a Black stranger into becoming her best friend so she doesn't lose touch with her roots. Ethan's manager signs me and helps me pitch the show to studios. It doesn't sell to any of them. But it does get me staffed on a series created by a novelist-turned-showrunner who likes it enough to give me a chance.

In Houston, my mother is hospitalized against her will again, but this time, upon her release, a bed turns out to be open in a good group home, where she will have her own room, twenty-four-hour assistance, and help getting and taking her medication. For the first few months, she refuses to see my grandmother or aunt when they visit, but gradually she settles in. My grandmother sends me a photo of the two of them standing next to each other on the green lawn of the group home; my mother is beaming.

Everything is going so well, and I'm so happy, that I decide to stop the antidepressants I've been on since her diagnosis. Shortly after, Ethan goes back to Guatemala for several weeks to finish his film, my time in the writer's room comes to an end, and, left to my own devices, I slip easily and all at once back into the abyss.

I USE THE MONEY I earned from writing for television to pay for a series of in-person ketamine therapy sessions. The sessions involve four weeks of regular therapy, followed by four weeks of injections, each of which is followed by a second therapy session done under the influence.

The therapist is young, sunny but grounded in a way that I don't find annoying, like a yoga teacher with legitimate medical knowledge and without the irritating unconditional optimism. In our earliest sessions, I'm plagued by the suspicion that I'm doing it wrong and she won't tell me, even though I'm the one paying her, exorbitantly, to be here, and even though I know consciously that it's not possible to do therapy wrong, because therapy doesn't have rules. It's this lack of rules, maybe, that is the problem.

"Who else made you feel like you were doing something wrong?" the therapist asks when I tell her this, and I think of the house in Riverside Terrace, of feeling terrified of the invisible trip wires that would detonate my mother's temper. My shoulders descend. I breathe.

When I tell her about my mother and how I feel as if I should have saved her, that I could have if I were a different person, she says, "That's the way a little kid thinks, and do you know why? Because it gives them the illusion of power. There is nothing you could have done."

I tell her about my discovery in Paris, my sense that everything is made up of smaller versions of itself branching out forever, and my fear that seeing this pattern everywhere means I'm experiencing apophenia. She says, Well, what if you're right? That would mean the Sarah you were when you were little is still in you now. She encourages me to speak to this smaller version of myself, to tell her she isn't wrong, that she can trust herself, that her mother is sick, that nothing happening to her is alright.

A doctor attends the following sessions to inject me with liquid ketamine. I listen to music for an hour while my body evaporates. I thought by undergoing therapy using a drug designed to remove its user from reality, I might better understand what my mother's day-to-day life is like. But that is not what happens. What happens feels specific to me.

Once the first trip begins, I am immediately twelve again, back in the car with my angry mother and my dogs, but this time Larry Bird is in the car with me and she is my protector and we are safe. I float down a tree-lined canyon as a single particle of self. I'm dead, but that's okay. I'm a branch spiraling off from my mother to start a new world. I swim in a waterfall where the water is a love whose abundance feels infinite.

In the therapy sessions that come after, the drug helps me take my stories apart and examine their contents so newness spills out. I come to understand that I've been trying to snap the pieces of my mother back into place, to build a whole I could eventually step back from and see my future reflected in. To build a picture of that far-off location where all her lives fit and break open and come back together. But now, I can see the pieces themselves, how they don't come together but lie on top of one another in layers.

Her anger was all-encompassing and brutal. She appeared at times to openly despise my grandmother, my aunt Tina, and me. She let herself be swallowed up by a rage that burned everything she ever touched. But she also gave me everything she had. But she also equipped me with all that I needed to leave and build the life I want. But also, somewhere, she is fourteen and in the car with Lance Blanks headed to the beach with the windows down, singing along to the radio, wearing striped socks and a denim jacket, surfing a hand through the air.

A LOCAL LOS ANGELES PRINTMAKER whose art revolves around fractals hires me to write an essay for her exhibition catalog about my obsession with trees. In researching the piece, I discover a book by a Duke engineering professor, Adrian Bejan, that posits that everything that exists came about as a manifestation of friction over a vast period of time. Lightning bolts happen where a build up of electricity must be discharged; animals evolve where water flows across land; trees sprout where more water sits in the ground than in the air.

One name for the shape this process creates is a Lichtenberg figure, and it is a figure one comes across again and again, in lightning, in rivers, in scars, and in trees, but also in vascular systems and the shapes of neurons and synapses, in the patterns of ice crystals on airplane windows, in the breaking off of torsos into arms, arms into hands, and hands into fingers: everything shaping itself according to the pathway that will allow it to gather fuel and grow most efficiently while expending the least amount of energy.

The shapes arise, according to Bejan, because of the Constructal Law, which "links the flow of rivers to the flow of cities and the flow of money"[38] by giving the patterns along which they expand a common structure. I'm thrilled with my discovery, and with the fact that what I thought was apophenia was, in fact, my noticing the signs of an already established rule.

A family tree follows this pattern, with many generations exploding outward from a single point. What's one more branch? I say to Ethan after therapy one day. Think about all the genes that fought their way from prehistory to the present through us. It doesn't seem fair to stop them here.

"You can't say you want a baby when you've always said the opposite before," Ethan says. But he says it thoughtfully. For my part, I do want a baby, but I do not want to suffer. We decide we will have a baby if we ever have a million dollars. We are not anywhere close to having a million dollars but we are, at the same time, further away from having negative dollars than we have ever been. For the past twelve years, together we've averaged a household income of about $36,000 a year, our lives subsidized almost entirely by the rent-controlled apartment we never expected to leave. But my first writing job led to another, and I've been working in television consistently. I have money put away for retirement. I have a brokerage account. We are saving for a house.

WALTER BENJAMIN COMMITTED SUICIDE BEFORE he could finish *The Arcades Project*. Crossing from Nazi-occupied France into Spain, he was turned back at the border because he did not have the exit visa required. His heart was weak, and he knew he wouldn't survive another attempt to leave. His final message reads, in part: "In a situation presenting no way out, I have no other choice but to make an end of it. It is in a small village in the Pyrenees, where no one knows me, that my life will come to a close."[39] Almost immediately after his death, from an overdose of morphine, the visa requirement was lifted. The other refugees traveling with him were allowed safe passage. It's possible that if Benjamin hadn't killed himself, he, too, would have made it to safety. It's also possible that the visa directive was only lifted because of the shocking nature of his passing.

An artist friend, Steffani Jemison, who understands my continued fascination with the story, compares Benjamin's death to the deaths of enslaved Africans who threw themselves off slave ships rather than be forcibly transferred to the New World. Both, she says, involve a decision to live and to complete your life on your own terms rather than on someone else's.

And in the end, Benjamin lived on his own terms as well. His friend Georges Bataille stored photocopies of Benjamin's extensive notes at the Bibliothèque Nationale in Paris until the war ended. In the 1950s, Gershom Scholem and Theodor Adorno published two volumes of his work with the assistance of Hannah Arendt. His French translator, Pierre Missac, helped make arrangements for publication of *The Arcades Project* in German and it was co-translated into English by my college professor, which was how it made its way to me. The life's work Benjamin died thinking of as a failure reached more readers than he could ever have imagined and changed the trajectory of critical thought.

...

IN 2022, DURING WHAT APPEARS to be a lull in the COVID-19 pandemic that has been raging now for two years, Ethan and I pass through Paris on our way back from a film festival in Reims. Paris is hotter than we expected, and we bicker on the street. I take him to see Benjamin's arcades, hoping he will be intrigued by the antique shops and the smoked glass ceilings stained from long-ago gas lamps, the mysterious light that makes the people who move through them look like phantoms. But he finds their kitsch overwhelming. "No offense," he says, as we pass the tourist trap wax museum at one passageway entrance, "but this is not really my thing."

We spend the afternoon drinking on the Canal Saint-Martin with friends of his from a French film distribution company. We have plans to fly home in the morning, but that night, at the hotel, I test positive for COVID. Due to the international travel rules at the time, I will not be allowed on the plane. We agree that Ethan will fly back alone to pick up the dog from the sitter. I sleep at the studio of a friend of a friend and then, still testing positive days later, move on to a stranger's fold-out couch in République, which I arrange via an internet forum for travelers, and where I languish alone in the dark.

Nearly a week in, when I wake up able to move again and finally testing negative, I decide to celebrate by drinking a glass of cold white wine alone in one of the cafés that line the canals. I choose one with two old men sitting at a small table arguing happily and, seized by the desire to insinuate myself into their conversation, I realize I miss Ethan.

While I'm sitting there, Ethan sends me a text—a photo of

him and the dog waking up—and I send a video back, turning my phone on the water, where the current pushes the river gently out to sea. On the sidewalk, a determined old woman pushes through a knot of tourists who fall backward as one in a kind of astonished wave. A girl on a bicycle whistles past and nearly hits me, bell dinging. People move up walkways, surge out of theaters, climb down into the metro, expand through tunnels, particles moving along a current, lives forking with every decision, every decision working in concert to deposit us here.

A rush of happiness passes through me and I let myself feel it without wondering when it will end. I ask myself a question, the question that occurred to the man in Bogotá: How do we know that what happens to us isn't good?

ACKNOWLEDGMENTS

THANK YOU TO LANCE BLANKS for seeing my mother in a way she could not see herself and for being kind enough to share your memories with me. The world is a much sadder place without you in it, and you are deeply missed.

Thank you to my literary agent, Claudia Ballard, and her assistant, Oma Naraine. Thank you to my editors, Adenike Olanrewaju and Jenny Xu. Thank you to Janet Byrne for copyedits and fact-checking. Thank you to Liz Velez. Thank you to my manager, Chris Davey, and to my TV agents, Alyssa Mahler and Amanda Hacohen.

Thank you to Ellen and Yuval. Thank you to Julie and everyone at Literary Affairs. Thank you to the *Los Angeles Review of Books*, especially Irene and Daya. Thank you to Patrick and Alissa, Frankie, Isaac, Elizabeth and Brian, Eddie and Adam, Rafa and Daveed and Ellen and Ben, for hiring me to work on your shows while I wrote this book.

Thank you to Yaddo, the Virginia Center for the Creative Arts, Ucross, Writers in the Schools, and the Ron Brown Scholar Program.

Thank you to Lou Mathews and everyone at NYU's MFA program, especially Deborah Landau, David Lipsky, and Ren Weschler. Thank you to Dan Alig, Mrs. George, Mrs. Costello, and Ms. Sims.

ACKNOWLEDGMENTS

Thank you to Steffani Jemison, Naima Lowe, Saaret E. Yoseph, Silas Munro, and everyone in the Breathing Room trajectory at Louis Place. Thank you also to J. Ryan Stradal, Steph Cha, Carmiel Banasky, Yvonne Zima, Rachel Kondo, Marya Spence, Lydia Conklin, Adam Dalva, and William Day Frank.

Thank you to Laura Hughes for inspiring me to move to France in high school, for pointing me toward Diderot's *Encyclopédie* in graduate school, and for your consistent warmth and intelligence at every stage of adulthood.

Thank you to the friends who, at various points in time, have all saved my life: Jen Hoguet, Aerin Snow, Will Bowling, Sarah Solemani, Aaliyah Williams, Alejandro Golding, and Kim Samek. Thank you to my half-siblings and my father, Stephen, and all of the Labries.

Thank you to the *good* therapists, especially Lauren Taus at In-bodied Life and Cynthia D'Anna. Thank you also to Pam Cantor and Laverne McKinnon.

Thank you to Rich and Jackie Lerner, for everything. I love you.

Thank you to my family for making me believe I could do anything, and thank you to Justin for showing me how.

NOTES

1. Franz Kafka, *The Diaries of Franz Kafka, 1910–1923* (New York: Schocken, 1988).
2. Daniel J. Siegel, *Mind: A Journey to the Heart of Being Human* (New York: W. W. Norton & Company, 2016).
3. Walter Benjamin's *Collected Works*, edited by Rolf Tiedemann and Hermann Schweppenhäuser with the collaboration of Theodor W. Adorno and Gershom Scholem (Frankfurt am Main: Suhrkamp Verlag, 1972–), Vol. V: *Das Passagen-Werk*, ed. Rolf Tiedemann (1982), 83 (A1, 1), cited by Susan Buck-Morss in *The Dialectics of Seeing: Walter Benjamin and the Arcades Project* (Cambridge, MA: MIT Press, 1989), 8.
4. Letter, Benjamin to Scholem, December 22, 1924, in *Briefe*, ed. Gershom Scholem and Theodor W. Adorno (Frankfurt am Main: Suhrkamp Verlag, 1966), Vol. 1, 366.
5. "Marshall Woman Becomes Member of Branch Staff," *Marshall News Messenger*, July 21, 1968.
6. Alex Poinsett, "Houston: Golden City of Opportunity," *Ebony*, July 1978.
7. Walter Benjamin and Gershom Scholem, *The Correspondence of Walter Benjamin and Gershom Scholem, 1932–1940*, ed. Gershom Scholem, trans. Gary Smith and André Lefevere (Cambridge, MA: Harvard University Press, 1992).
8. Walter Benjamin, *Illuminations*, ed. Hannah Arendt, trans. Harry Zohn (New York: Schocken, 2007), 19.
9. I'm taking some liberties here. This quote is attributed to Monty Williams, who coached the Phoenix Suns, and as far as I can tell, his saying it is not documented before 2019.
10. Dr. Helen Grusd cited in Sarah Haufrect, "I Loved, Lived with, and

Lost My Mother to Borderline Personality Disorder," Salon.com, February 28, 2016, https://www.salon.com/2016/02/28/i_loved_lived _with_and_lost_my_mother_to_borderline_personality_disorder/.

11. Jennifer Egan quoted in Alexandra Schwartz, "Jennifer Egan's Travels Through Time," *The New Yorker*, October 9, 2017, https://www .newyorker.com/magazine/2017/10/16/jennifer-egans-travels-through -time.

12. Ethan Watters, *Crazy Like Us: The Globalization of the American Psyche* (New York: Free Press, 2011), e-book.

13. Juli McGruder cited in Watters, *Crazy Like Us*, 165.

14. Walter Benjamin, *The Arcades Project*, ed. Rolf Tiedemann, trans. Howard Eiland and Kevin McLaughlin (Cambridge, MA: Belknap Press of Harvard University Press, 1999), 26.

15. Walter Benjamin, "Theses on the Philosophy of History," in Benjamin, *Illuminations*, 12, 257.

16. Gillian B. White, "How Black Middle-Class Kids Become Poor Adults," *Atlantic*, January 19, 2015, https://www.theatlantic.com/business /archive/2015/01/how-black-middle-class-kids-become-black-lower -class-adults/384613/; Tracy Jan, "White Families Have Nearly 10 Times the Net Worth of Black Families. And the Gap Is Growing," *Washington Post*, September 28, 2017, https://www.washingtonpost .com/news/wonk/wp/2017/09/28/black-and-hispanic-families-are -making-more-money-but-they-still-lag-far-behind-whites/.

17. Walter Benjamin, "Franz Kafka: On the 10th Anniversary of his Death," in Benjamin, *Illuminations*, 116.

18. Resmaa Menakem, *My Grandmother's Hands* (Nevada: Central Recovery Press, 2017), e-book.

19. Christine Ann Lawson, *Understanding the Borderline Mother* (New Jersey: Jason Aronson, 2000), 44–45.

20. James Baldwin, *Notes of a Native Son* (New York: Beacon Press, 1955), 88, 96, 102, 113.

21. James Baldwin, 1961 radio interview, WBAI, New York, https://www .youtube.com/watch?v=jNpitdJSXWY.

22. Jonathan M. Metzl, *The Protest Psychosis* (Boston: Beacon Press, 2009), ix, 30.

23. Arrah Evarts, "Dementia Precox in the Colored Race," *Psychoanalytic Review* 1, no. 4 (1914): 388–403; cited in Metzl, *The Protest Psychosis*, 31. I was first made aware of Evarts's work thanks to the book *Body Work* by Melissa Febos.

24. E. Franklin Frazier, "The Pathology of Race Prejudice," *Forum* 77, no. 6 (June 1927): 856–62.

25. Sigmund Freud, "Constructions in Analysis," in *The Standard Edition of the Complete Psychological Works of Sigmund Freud*, trans. James Strachey, Vol. XXIII (London: Hogarth Press, 1937–39), 269.

26. Preston Lauterbach, "Memphis Burning," *Places Journal*, March 2016, https://placesjournal.org/article/memphis-burning/?cn-reloaded=1.

27. Benjamin and Scholem, *The Correspondence of Walter Benjamin and Gershom Scholem, 1932–1940*.

28. Gershom Scholem, *Walter Benjamin: The Story of a Friendship* (New York: New York Review Books, 2012), e-book.

29. Amy Hempel, *Reasons to Live* (New York: HarperCollins, 1985), 98.

30. Franz Kafka, *The Zürau Aphorisms*, trans. Michael Hofmann (New York: Schocken, 2006), note 93, 91.

31. Arcades Project cited by Esther Leslie in "Ruin and Rubble in the Arcades," in *Walter Benjamin and the Arcades Project*, ed. Beatrice Hanssen (New York: Continuum, 2006), 101.

32. James Baldwin, *The Fire Next Time* (New York: Modern Library, 1995), 91–92.

33. Mark Swed, "Review: From 19th Century Memphis to Modern-Day L.A.: Master Chorale Time-Travels Through 'Dreams of the New World,'" *Los Angeles Times*, May 14, 2018.

34. *The Correspondence of Walter Benjamin and Gershom Scholem, 1932–1940*, cited in Leland de la Durantaye, "Sedan Chairs and Turtles," *London Review of Books*, November 21, 2013, https://www.lrb.co.uk/the-paper/v35/n22/leland-de-la-durantaye/sedan-chairs-and-turtles; Sarah LaBrie, "Theodor Adorno, Letters to Walter Benjamin," *New Left Review* 1/81, Sept./Oct. 1973, https://newleftreview.org/issues/i81/articles/14?token=1HHpyg6hpM0t.

35. Howard Eiland and Michael W. Jennings, *Walter Benjamin: A Critical Life* (Cambridge: Harvard University Press, 2016), Kindle edition, 623–624.

36. Adam Kirsch, "The Philosopher Stoned," *The New Yorker*, August 21, 2006.
37. Leo Tolstoy, *War and Peace*, trans. Louise and Aylmer Maude (Oxford: Oxford University Press, 1952).
38. Adrian Bejan, *Design in Nature: How the Constructal Law Governs Evolution in Biology, Physics, Technology, and Social Organizations* (New York: Anchor, 2018).
39. Walter Benjamin, *The Arcades Project*, ed. Rolf Tiedemann, trans. Howard Eiland and Kevin McLaughlin (Cambridge, MA: Belknap Press of Harvard University Press, 1999), 953.

ABOUT THE AUTHOR

SARAH LABRIE is a writer from Houston, Texas. Her libretti have been performed at Walt Disney Concert Hall and her fiction has appeared in *Guernica*, *The Literary Review*, and the *Los Angeles Review of Books*. She has held residencies at Yaddo, Ucross, and the Virginia Center for the Creative Arts. She lives in Los Angeles, where she has written for television shows, including *Minx* (Starz), *Blindspotting* (Starz), *Made for Love* (MAX), and *Love, Victor* (Hulu). She holds an MFA from NYU, where she was a Writers in the Public Schools Fellow.